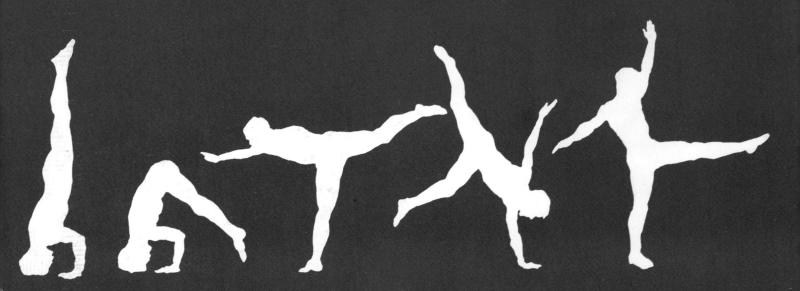

THE COMPLETE
HEAD TO TOE
EXERCISE BOOK
Get fitter ~ feel better

CHARTWELL
BOOKS, INC.

Edited by Linda Fox

Published by Chartwell Books, Inc.
a Division of Book Sales, Inc.
110 Enterprise Avenue
Secaucus, New Jersey

Printed and bound in Hong Kong by Dai Nippon Printing Company

ISBN 0-89009-752-6

Introduction

Are you physically fit? Can you indulge in a sudden burst of strenuous activity without getting aches and pains? Just try the fitness test in the first chapter of this book and you'll soon find out!

Even if you know you're really out of condition, don't worry. With this book of specially designed courses for both men and women you can choose your own way to head-to-toe fitness. Why join expensive classes when you can exercise in comfort at home from these simple step-by-step programmes? Take it at your own pace, concentrate on the exercises that benefit you most, exercise regularly — and you'll soon be on the way to total fitness.

The Complete Head to Toe Exercise Book is a comprehensive manual for everyone who wants to enjoy the rewards that come with regular exercise. And these rewards are well worth the effort: a feeling of vitality and well-being, a firm and supple shape, and glowing health that other people will envy. Most people today exercise their minds more than they exercise their bodies — and it shows! A session of simple exercises once a day is one of the best ways to relax. And with this book you can exercise when it suits you: in the morning to get set up for the day, or in the evening to induce a pleasant feeling of tiredness and a good night's sleep. You can exercise on your own, or get the whole family to join in. No wonder more and more people are realizing that exercise and recreation lead to a healthier and fuller life.

Try the six part Fitness course, just thirty minutes a day, specially designed for busy people. Trim away your unwanted bulges with simple exercises for all the most common figure faults. Take a home course in Gymnastics, or even Weightlifting. Along with all these fully-illustrated courses you will find a wealth of sensible information on keeping fit, such as why your body needs exercise, and the importance of combining exercise with correct diet, particularly if you want to lose weight. Plus a complete run-down of all the sports and recreations you can enjoy in your leisure time: how they will benefit your health, how expensive they are in terms of equipment, and the level of skill required. You don't need to be a competitive sportsman to enjoy walking, jogging or swimming. But there are plenty of more organized sports like football, golf, sailing or squash — and it's a great way to meet people.

So don't delay, make a resolution today to get fit and stay fit. Exercising the Head-to-Toe way isn't hard work at all — you'll enjoy it, and you'll reap all the benefits of head-to-toe health.

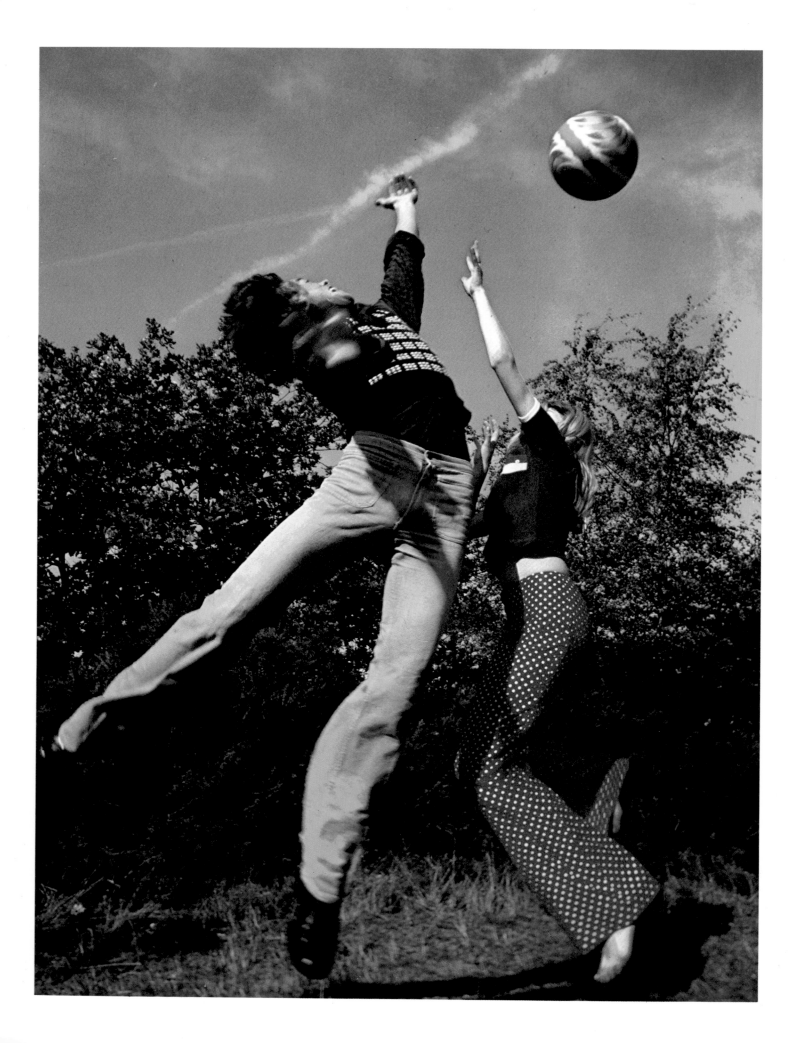

Contents

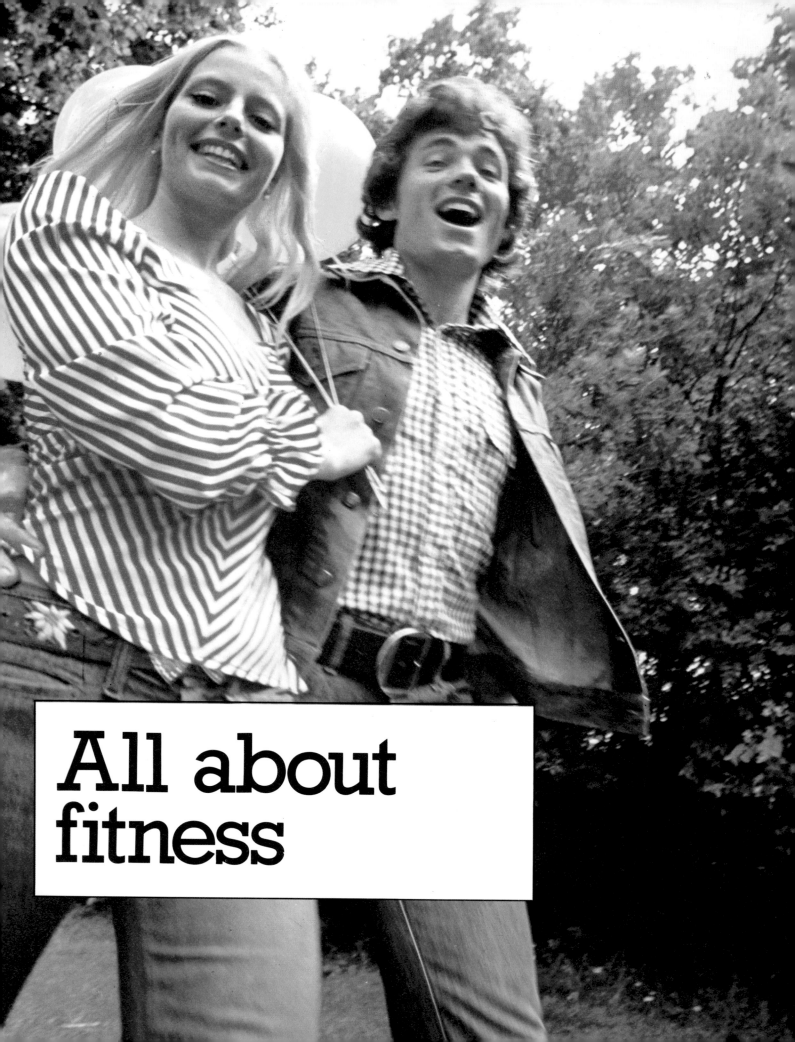

All about
fitness

Are You Physically Fit?

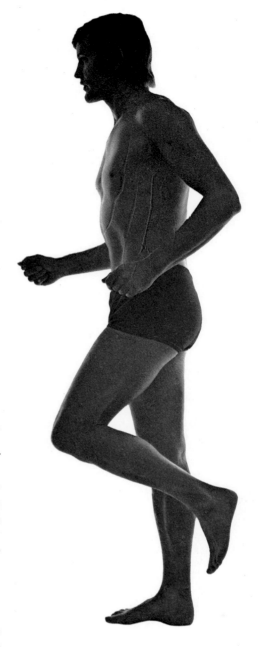

If you can run for a bus without getting breathless, if you can carry a heavy shopping bag without straining, if you can climb up several flights of stairs without your legs aching, then you probably think you are physically fit. But you could be wrong.

Physical fitness is not the ability to perform specific feats. It is the condition of your overall physiological, biochemical and mental state. If you are physically fit you can effectively work, play, resist chronic disease and meet the demands which are constantly made upon you.

Everyone has a unique physical potential. It is often difficult to fulfil this potential, but once you have, your pleasures and abilities will be experienced at their height. Your life will be richer.

Despite the breathless dash for the bus or train, most of us still maintain we are reasonably fit. But are we? Now you can find out how fit you really are with a simple but comprehensive test.

And, as you grow older and the conditions of your life change, you will continue to react in the most efficient way.

But how can you tell if you are physically fit?

To begin with, isolated performances do not give a true indication of physical fitness. Whether or not you can touch your toes, for example, is of little significance. If the way your bones are put together—the relative lengths of legs to trunk to arms—makes it mechanically impossible for you to touch your toes, you may still be more fit than a person who can touch his toes without difficulty. Nor is the ability to lift heavy weights a sound criterion of physical fitness. Many strong men are unfit, despite their muscular power.

To decide if you are physically fit, you have to look at your body, at your performance and at your response to stress and to physical exertion. Each person is different and the aim is to discover whether you have reached your individual potential of physical fitness. You may be unfit but still skilled enough at a sport to perform better than someone who is fit.

The overall quality of your life is not,

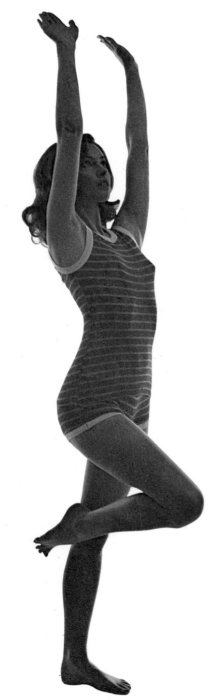

however, measured by an isolated comparison. If you lift a heavier weight than the next person, and pull a muscle while he remains happily composed, you will have won a battle but lost the war. Competition with regard to fitness is not the competition of the sports field—it is a struggle against your own lack of fitness.

The human body is an extremely efficient physiological and biochemical machine. But it is also subject to physical laws, some of them of great subtlety. And if those laws are broken the penalties are severe. On the other hand, the body can stand a lot of abuse. The potential for getting the most from life is there for the vast majority of people—providing they are physically fit.

If you are fit you will be able to work and play to the full, and when you become tired you will be able to relax. Sleep will restore your vigour. A criterion of your own state of fitness, therefore, is simply the answer to this question: Can you work and play as hard as you wish and get the rest you want so that you eagerly face the challenges of another day? If your honest answer is no, the demands made upon you are clearly greater than your ability to cope, and the strain is making inroads upon your physical and emotional capacity.

If you are overweight, your fitness will inevitably be lower than it would otherwise be. It is possible to be marginally overweight and still be fit in terms of what you can achieve physically and in your general vitality. Nevertheless, in most cases overweight indicates a reduced fitness standard. In ascertaining your physical fitness, you should make it a priority to check your weight.

The measurement of fitness is complex. Ideally, you want to know the extent of your endurance, your strength, your co-ordination and the speed with which you can recover from exertion. You should not need to slump gratefully into a seat after running for a bus.

It would be useful if it were possible to take a series of scientific measurements and, on their basis, determine if a particular person were as fit as could be expected. It can be determined if something is seriously wrong with a person—if, for example, he or she has high blood pressure or a slow recovery rate after physical exercise. But, because of great physical variations, it is very difficult by these means to ascertain an individual's general level of fitness or to compare his level with that of someone else.

Physical fitness can most effectively be determined by measuring the responses of the body to specific activities. The reactions measured are usually the change in heart beat and blood pressure. The pulse rate, which is the measurement of how many times a minute the heart beats, can disclose a great deal about physical fitness.

People who are physically fit can perform the same amount of work with less effort than those who are unfit. Thus, a

How Fit Are You?

These simple exercises will help you assess your own physical fitness. They will also indicate the areas in which your weaknesses lie.

It is best if you do these exercises when you are rested and relaxed. If you feel fatigued while you are doing them stop immediately and rest. If you have recently been ill, consult your doctor before beginning.

For some of these exercises you will need a watch with a second hand to measure your pulse rate. To take your pulse, press the tips of the first and second fingers of your right hand lightly on the inner wrist, below the thumb, of the left hand. Count the number of pulsations of the artery for the required length of time.

Breathing

1 Stand in a relaxed position, your feet apart and your arms at your sides. Take a deep breath. Exhale. Inhale deeply and hold your breath. Score one point if you can hold it for 45 seconds or more.

2 Inhale deeply and measure your chest around the rib cage with a tape measure. Exhale and measure your chest again. If the difference is three and a half inches or more, if you are a man, and two and a half inches or more, if you are a woman, score one point.

Endurance

Immediately after completing each of the following exercises, count your pulse rate for 15 seconds. Score one point for a rate of 32 beats or less. Rest for five minutes after each exercise.

3 Standing in one place, jump up and down on your toes 20 times in 30 seconds. Try to jump to a count of one, two, three. Bend your knees between each jump. Your toes should be four to five inches from the ground at the top of your jump.

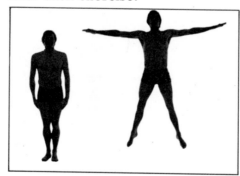

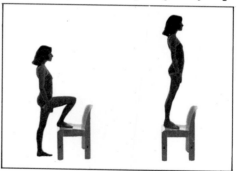

4 Starting with your legs together in a standing position and your arms at your sides, raise your arms to shoulder height and, at the same time, jump to spread legs at least 15 inches apart. Repeat 25 times in 30 seconds.

5 Step up and down on a sturdy chair which has a seat about 18 inches from the ground. Repeat 24 times in one minute. Step up with your right leg first for 12 steps, and with your left leg for the remaining steps.

Strength

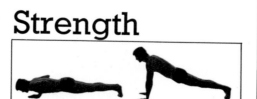

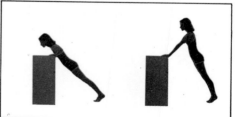

6 Try to do press-ups. To do press-ups, men should lie face-down on the floor. Place both hands on the floor, palms down, in line with and about three inches from your shoulders. Keeping your back straight, raise your body by straightening your arms. Women should do this exercise by leaning against a firmly-placed table, at a 45-degree angle with the floor, and pushing up from the shoulders. Score one point if you complete 10.

7 Lie on your back, with your feet placed against the underside of some immovable object, such as a bed or the rung of a table. Sit up, as slowly as possible, with your arms extended in front of you. Score one point if you can sit up 10 times.

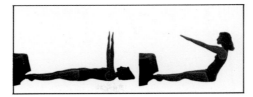

8 Stand on your toes, arms extended in front of you, with your back against a wall. Bend your legs slowly to a squatting position, keeping your back against the wall. Straighten your legs to resume the original position. Score one point if you can do this 10 times.

Balance and Suppleness

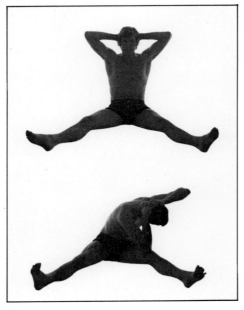

9 Balance on your right leg. Bend forwards slowly from the waist, raising your arms out to the sides, and lifting your left leg back as high as possible. Repeat, balancing on the left leg. Score one point if you can hold each position for 10 seconds.

10 Sit on the floor with your back straight and your legs apart, so that they form two sides of a triangle whose sides are of equal length. With your hands clasped behind your head, bend forward slowly. Try to touch your left knee with your right elbow, and then your right knee with your left elbow. Score one point if you can complete both movements successfully. It is important that you do not strain.

Speed and Co-ordination

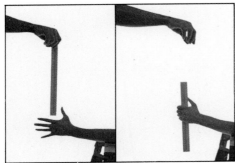

11 Place your arm on a table with your hand extending over the edge. Now ask a friend to hold a 12-inch ruler at its top, so that the bottom is close to your hand. As he releases the ruler, try to catch it. Score one point if you catch the ruler two out of three times.

12 Score one point if you can skip with a rope, continuously, for 30 skips.

The maximum score on this test is 12 points. A score of over eight points is good. If you have reached eight points or more, however, you should not conclude that this is the highest level of fitness you can achieve. There is virtually no upper limit to physical fitness. If you have achieved such a score, and are below 30 years old, it is important to remember that your level of physical fitness may deteriorate as you grow older unless you take steps to maintain it.

A score of under five points, on the other hand, shows that you need to take immediate measures to become more physically fit. If you have scored between five and eight points, there is still good reason for you to start to raise the level of your fitness.

fit person doing moderate work will usually have a heart rate of about 120 beats per minute, while an unfit person doing the same work will score upwards of 160. Furthermore, the unfit person's heart takes longer to return to its normal rate, which is about 72 beats per minute.

There are tests which use these techniques in a simple way and which will give you a fairly reliable indication of your fitness. If you are seriously unfit, they will reveal this in a few moments. If you are reasonably fit you should be able to perform most of the tests successfully. This does not mean, of course, that you have attained your peak of fitness. You may well be far below your best.

In considering your score on this or any fitness test, it is important that you remember that it can be no more than a general guide. If you have scored a high rating, this should spur you on to see just how fit you can get. The middle rating scores should at least encourage you to try to achieve a higher one. Low scoring means that you really should start to do something about becoming fit.

Irrespective of your score, if you smoke and inhale more than 15 cigarettes a day, you can anticipate declining fitness—if you continue to smoke. You will also lessen your fitness if you drink alcohol immoderately.

We still do not know all there is to know about fitness. There is much to be learned about the effects of intense physical exercise and why athletic training makes fatigue less likely. But it has been established that lack of exercise results in impaired strength, endurance and performance. In particular, the unexercised body requires a greater time to recover from exertion.

We know, too, that lessened physical fitness with age is not only related to the aging process. The decrease in physical fitness in men and women between the ages of 30 and 50 years old is usually the result of neglect. There is no need for anyone to become unfit as they grow older—and it is possible to restore physical fitness or to raise it to higher levels.

Exercise is the great key to fitness. The body's vitality declines as the result of a sedentary and stressful life, one very often combined with bad eating habits. Muscles, whether they are the biceps or the heart, become less efficient if they are not sufficiently used. While the physiological mechanism may not be completely understood, there is no doubt that the well-exercised person, who eats a well-balanced diet, will have the strength and energy that comes with physical fitness.

The first step is to assess just how fit, or unfit, you are. If this test shows that you are not as fit as you might be, start exercising today. And continue to test yourself every month. You will be impressed by the improvement. Physical fitness is like a crisp, juicy apple. You don't know how good it is until you bite into it.

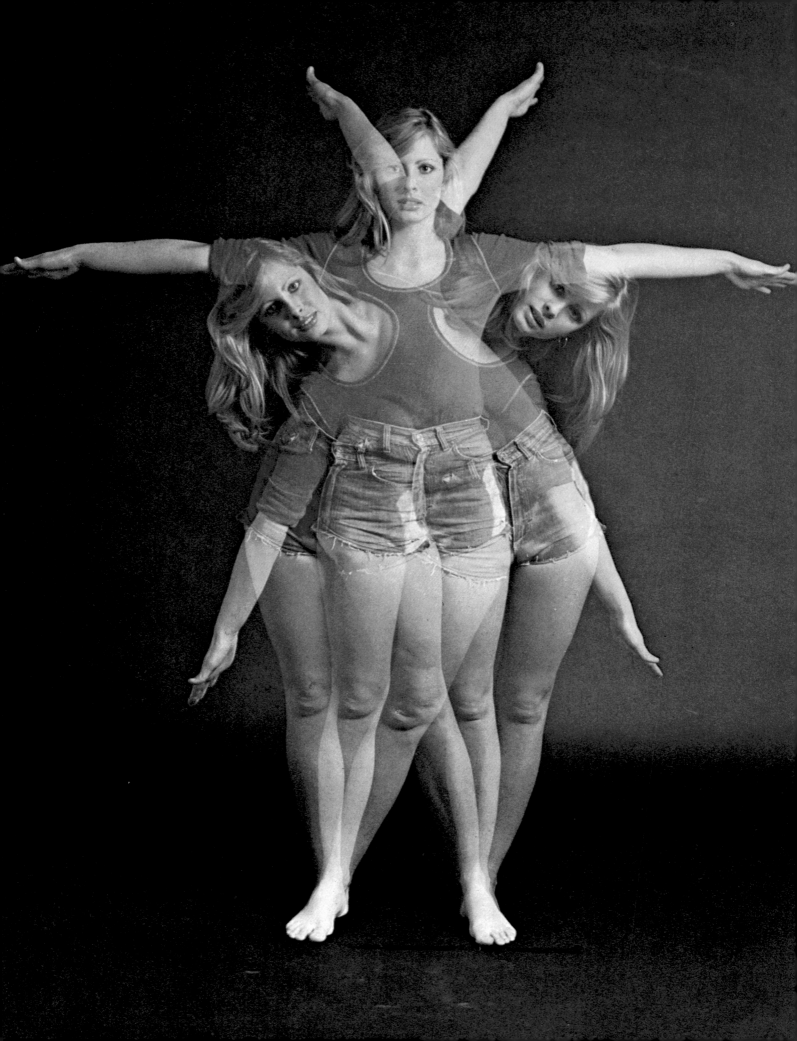

Can Exercise Make You Slim?

Losing weight should present a simple equation—you can either keep up the same amount of exercise but eat less, or you can increase your output of energy while maintaining your intake of food.

It sounds easy enough. But a closer look at the effort involved in losing a significant amount of weight, and losing it quickly, through exercise alone can be daunting. The statistics are certainly discouraging. To lose one pound of fat you would have to walk at least 30 miles. To compensate for a cheese sandwich you would have to play squash for one hour. Swimming the English Channel demands an energy outlay of up to 12,000 Calories, or three and a half pounds of body fat. And even an extra spoonful of sugar in your tea or coffee requires a brisk half-mile walk, or the excess could add up to an overload of about 15 pounds at the end of a year.

So, for the person who wants to lose weight, just how much use is exercise?

First, it must be asked whether it is possible to lose weight without exercising at all. Recent medical research has shown that, under careful supervision, it is possible to lose unwanted fat without even lifting a finger.

Obese people (the usual definition of obese is 20 per cent or more heavier than normal for a particular height, age and sex) have been kept in hospital for long periods of time on a starvation diet of water, supplemented only by the vitamins and minerals that the body needs for survival. Under these conditions it has been shown that people can lose as much as five pounds a week if they weigh 280 pounds or more, and proportionately less if they are lighter. In less severe cases, supervised dieting on 800 to 1,000 Calories a day almost always results in a steady average reduction of three pounds a week. In all these cases, the men and women were confined to hospital and the weight loss was achieved without any exercise at all.

The prevailing medical opinion today is that the effective way to lose weight, if this is what becoming slim basically means, is to consume fewer calories. Not only is it so much easier to give up a spoonful of sugar rather than to walk half a mile, but for anyone who wants to lose 15 pounds or more in a fairly short time there are not enough hours in the day for the necessary exercise, even if the inclination is there.

But although exercise alone will not result in instant weight loss, Dr. John Durnin, author of *Energy, Work and Leisure* and a physiologist who has carried out many studies on human energy expenditure, suggests that it is highly likely that today most overweight people have become fat not because they eat too much, but because they exercise too little. As a result of modern technological advances, the increasing numbers of cars and labour-saving machines and gadgets means that men and women use their muscles less and less in doing their jobs and in getting from place to place. Television, too, contributes to the process by luring people away from more active entertainment. And, while the work-load has shrunk, food still keeps coming in the same-sized helpings.

Once a person has put on weight, his or her movements tend to slow down to the pace of other fat people. In a test conducted in Philadelphia, groups of fat and slim people, of the same sex and similar social backgrounds and occupations, were each given a pedometer to wear all day for up to two weeks to measure how many miles a day they walked. The results showed that in nearly every case the thinner people covered about twice the distance of the overweight group.

The effects of such sluggish activity are, of course, cumulative. Exercise, therefore, can be of great value in preventing any increase in weight, and in keeping the body lively and supple.

Exercise also provides an excellent complementary programme if you are on a low-calorie diet. Exercise can help you to lose inches rather than weight, and attain or retain a more attractive shape. If you cut down your food and step up your exercise, you speed up the slimming process and improve your appearance

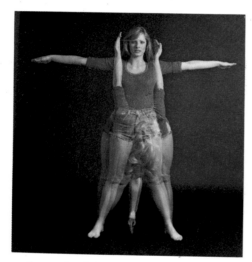

and your health at the same time.

The rate of weight loss is a vital factor for most people who want to slim. They are not content with losing a pound or so a month—the amount lost by walking briskly for half an hour each day while maintaining the same food intake. But to maintain the same diet and reach their target of two or three pounds weight loss a week would require a deficit of about 1,000 Calories a day—a proportion that would entail a degree of physical activity way beyond most people. To lose that amount of weight you would have to swim three hours a day, seven days a week.

The answer, then, is a compromise: cutting down the intake of calories and disposing of the surplus energy stored in the body by moderate, regular exercise.

The fat in your body is not solid like a lump of butter or the fat on a piece of raw meat. The heat of the body keeps it in liquid form so that it is more like oil. This liquid fat is stored in minute fat-deposit cells, where it stays until (if ever) it is called upon to supply the body with reserve energy. If you eat more food than your body uses up in energy, the excess is hoarded. Fresh stores of oil are forced into each cell so that the cells gradually swell up.

It helps to understand this if you imagine that a slim person has fat cells rather like bunches of small grapes. If the body puts on weight, these cells increase in size until they become like

luscious dessert grapes. The only way to reduce the size of the large fat cells is to cut down on the food supply or increase activity. In either case the body is forced to draw on its reserves of fat. The cells will then gradually shrink back to normal. These fat-deposit cells, however, are only tapped by the body as a last resort. For the normal functioning of the muscles, the body usually uses up energy in the form of glucose which is found in the blood. If this runs out the muscles have to draw on their own source of glycogen and, only when the muscles require still more fuel, are the stores of energy in the adipose (fat) tissue drawn upon.

There is no doubt that you can lose both weight and inches if you increase your exercise without eating more food. However, there are two drawbacks. The first is that your body can only cope with sudden bouts of heavy physical exercise if it is fit enough to do so and has worked up to it gradually through milder forms of exertion. If you are overweight it is almost certain that you are also physically out of condition, and any sudden demands would put a heavy strain on your muscles, your joints and your heart. The second difficulty is that if you want to lose a large amount of weight you will probably have neither the stamina nor the time to burn up sufficient calories.

Squash, a game that is rapidly gaining popularity throughout the world, and particularly in Britain and Australia, is a good example. It is a strenuous and energetic game and uses up more calories per minute than almost any other sport. But although it can consume calories at the rate of over 10 a minute, or

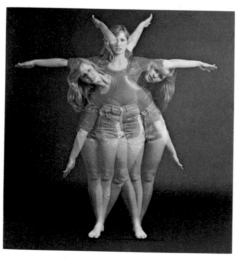

600 an hour, it cannot be played for long periods of time. Anyone who was out of condition and played squash for 30 minutes would be taking an enormous health risk.

Most experts point out that it is the more moderate types of exercise that can be pursued for longer periods of time that will ultimately be the most effective. It is a great temptation to believe that a heavy work-out which leaves you sweat-

ing and tired must have had the desired effect. But losing weight by exercising is a gradual, even process. Extra energy spent walking, for example, could be divided up throughout the day. A 20-minute walk to the station or to work in the morning and back again at night would, over the course of several weeks, be much more rewarding than a few hectic sessions of squash, tennis or swimming.

The results of slimming through

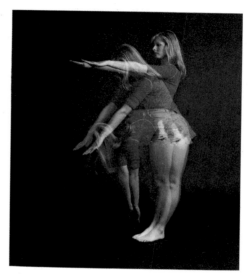

moderate exercise are not dramatic over a short time. But in the same way that eating a quarter of a pound of butter a week more than you use up in energy can make you one pound heavier at the end of a month, an hour's brisk walk each day could reduce your weight by 10 pounds at the end of a year. And you would still be eating the way you did before. Any additional sport or exercise, of course, provides a bonus—more pounds and inches lost.

The best form of exercise for you depends to a large extent on your own particular way of life. The most important thing is that you should exercise regularly, so your choice should be tailored to fit your circumstances. Most office workers, for example, are unfit. Many of them are overweight, and many of them do not have enough time to devote to full-scale exercise to keep in good shape.

Al Murray, a physiotherapist and a former British Olympic coach who runs a gymnasium in London, maintains that controlled exercise, under supervision, for only 15 minutes three times a week, can produce a significant improvement in a man's general fitness. If this exercise is increased to four times a week a man of 25 years old who is about 15 pounds overweight could lose up to 10 pounds in six weeks. He could possibly lose this amount of weight in four weeks if his increased fitness significantly speeds up his daily output of energy, as it usually does. This is only true, of course, if he eats no more than he did before he began exercising. This can demand will-power if he feels somehow that extra exercise should entitle him to consume more food.

Some people do claim that they get hungrier and eat more if they exercise. This increased hunger, which is often psychological, tends to be temporary. And it must be ignored if the benefits of exercise are to be reflected on the tape measure.

While the time involved in exercise is an important factor for most people, so frequently is space. Many people live in fairly small rooms that are too cramped to encourage the psychological and physical freedom of exercise. For those who prefer to exercise at home, rather than in a gym, some types of exercise will be better than others.

A few years ago, jogging swept the United States as an exercise primarily aimed at increasing the efficiency of the heart and muscles, but also as an attack on unwanted weight. Medical research has shown that this type of exercise was the most effective way of improving cardio-vascular (heart and lung) efficiency in a short period of time. And while jogging is of greater all-round benefit if it is carried out in the fresh air of the country, jogging or running on the spot can use up a significant amount of calories and can be achieved in an area no larger than you use to stand up in.

Another good all-round exercise, one that burns up the calories even faster than jogging, is rope-skipping. It is no coincidence that boxers use it as one of the major elements of their training, but it will probably appeal more to women than men. In tests carried out in Wash-

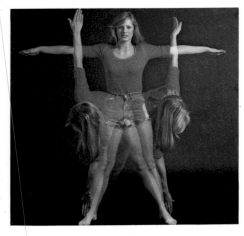

ington by John A. Baker, in 1968, it was found that 10 minutes of rope-skipping was as effective for cardio-vascular efficiency as 30 minutes of jogging. As with every other kind of strenuous physical activity, however, it should be embarked on gently so that the heart is not overtaxed. You should start for one or two minutes each day, doing a slow skip of 80 to 100 turns of the rope a minute.

The faster you do any physical activity, of course, the more calories you burn up. If you find it difficult to gauge just how much exercise you should aim to do without overtaxing yourself, you

can get an indication from various schedules, including the one produced by the Royal Canadian Air Force. A daily exercise programme is worked out for both men and women, giving recommendations for minimum and maximum performance targets for different age groups.

People who follow such a course of exercises, or are persistent with yoga,

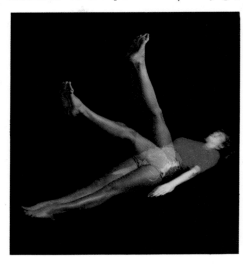

find that their bodies gradually become more shapely. Some lose weight, some don't, but they all lose inches and gain better proportions. Slimming, after all, is not necessarily the same as losing weight. Exercise can often result in staying the same weight and looking better and thinner.

Some people, particularly women, want to lose weight in specific areas. While exercise is more efficient in this respect than is dieting, most experts on physical training do not believe in attacking the "target area" in isolation. They feel it is better to first get the body into a healthy condition, and then to concentrate on the problem with special exercises.

It should be remembered, however, that your body can only be trimmed within the framework of your own bone structure. The odd inch or two, if it is excess fat, can be removed, but you cannot change your basic body shape. A girl who has a narrow torso and large hips, for example, will die of starvation before she becomes a slim, willowy reed. And a rounded, strongly endomorphic-type man will never become a Tarzan, despite all the exercise and will in the world. Spot-reduction can be achieved by concentrating the physical activity on the muscles in the area concerned, but the basic shape will remain the same.

A fear of building up muscles puts many people off the idea of exercise. But their worries are unjustified. A healthy, well-formed muscle is a good shape, compact but not fat. To get large, over-developed muscles you would have to devote several hours a day to slowly and painfully building them up from every angle through a series of varied exer-

cises. Nor does muscle turn to fat once you stop any moderate and sensible activity. Exercise tones muscle up, and even if you stop physical activity completely the muscle merely returns to its untoned state.

Another fact that can be daunting is that exercise is only effective in keeping your body in good shape if you keep it up. You certainly won't look any worse after giving up exercise than you did before you started, and it may take a little time for your body to slip back to its original sluggishness, but it will get there in the end.

If you have lost weight as a result of strict dieting and increased exercise and then want to continue on a maintenance diet alone, you can do so successfully—provided you sustain the necessary balance of energy between intake and expenditure. Once you have developed the habit of regular physical activity, however, it is a pity to lapse back into a lazy way of life, losing your hard-earned suppleness. It may help to remember that if you continue with a little regular exercise your maintenance diet can afford to be that much richer—without any extra pounds creeping back.

In the complicated debate about exercise and diet, you are left with several choices, not all of them easy. It has now been proved that weight can be lost without exercising—but to lose a significant amount is a slow, painful business requiring immense will-power and self-discipline. On the other side of the argument, it is possible to lose weight and get thinner through exercise while retaining the same intake of food. But for exercise to be effective it means devoting an unrealistic amount of time to the problem.

The answer lies somewhere in the middle. A combination of dieting and

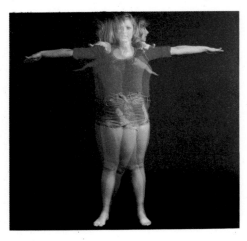

exercise is the only sure way to slim. The type and severity of the diet and the intensity and regularity of the exercise will depend on the extent of the problem. But if you are overweight, the first step should not be a difficult choice. You must use diet and exercise together to derive the full benefits of both and become a healthier and livelier person.

What Happens When

With powerful movements of your arms and legs, you swim a length of the pool. Exerting careful coordination and control, you swing your golf club back and bring it down punishingly on the ball, driving it with one bounce onto the green. Dog at heel, you stroll across the park. Dedicated and determined, you embark on your early morning exercise programme. On a fine summer day, you get out your bicycle and set off for an afternoon's ride. But what happens when you exercise?

The human body is an intricate mechanical system of bone, muscle, joint and tendon, and in every form of exercise, from golf to swimming, these combine in action, superbly coordinated by nervous messages. Bones give strength, support and form to the body. They meet at joints, which act like hinges to allow relative movement between the bones. Every voluntary movement is produced by the contraction of muscles, which span one or more joints and are attached to the bones by strong tendons.

In this way, the body acts rather like a complex system of levers. Its action is quite simple in principle, and yet behind even the simplest movement is an intricate web of biochemical and physiological activity. These systems, perfected in their role by evolution, are brought into play by every exercise regime.

Obviously, different forms of exercise involve different muscles, and the amount of effort involved also varies. An Olympic sprinter works harder than a man walking his dog, but virtually the same set of muscles and joints are involved. On the other hand, a series of press-ups or push-ups obviously exercises a different set of muscles and joints from those which are exercised when riding a bicycle. But the differences are all of degree and emphasis. They are not differences of principle.

The prime centres of activity in all forms of exercise are, of course, the muscles. Muscles vary in size and shape from flat sheets, like those which form the abdominal walls, to the tapering, spindle-shaped muscles of the arms and legs. Yet all muscles are formed from the same basic units—bundles of hair-like muscle fibres. Under a powerful microscope these fibres are seen to consist of large numbers of finer fibres called myofibrils. And within these are two kinds of filaments whose activity forms the basis of all muscular contraction.

When a muscle fibre is stimulated by a nerve signal, chemical changes within it cause one type of filament to slide into the other thicker filament with what is rather like a chemical ratchet action. The result is a shortening of the myo-fibrils and, in turn, a shortening of the muscle fibre.

The action of the whole muscle depends on the action of its individual fibres. In a maximum contraction, like that involved in the massive effort of a weightlifter, every available muscle fibre shortens. In a weak contraction, as in the gentle touch of a lover, only a few muscle fibres shorten. This is because individual muscle fibres act on an all-or-nothing principle—they either contract to their maximum possible extent or not at all. As they shorten, muscle fibres thicken, as can be seen whenever someone shows off the size of his biceps.

When a movement is reversed the muscle concerned does not reverse its action and push. The only active movement a muscle can make is to pull. Reversing the action requires the contraction of another muscle, the so-called antagonist. This at the same time stretches the first muscle, the synergist, back to its original length. In this way, the muscles at the front of the thigh, pulling across the knee joint, straighten

Despite the difference in effort, an Olympic sprinter and a man taking his dog for a walk employ the same sets of muscles and joints.

the leg, while those at the back bend it. In cycling, for example, these two sets of muscles act alternately.

Every muscle in the body has one or more antagonists. The action and counteraction between them is of supreme importance in all forms of exercise and sport, for it is the mechanism by which bodily movements are smoothed, controlled and coordinated. In this way, gentle action of the triceps muscle at the back of the upper arm steadies the counteraction of the biceps, and vice versa. A movement produced by a single muscle alone, without slight, progressive resistance from its antagonist, is jerky, like that of a clockwork manikin. A complex series of unconscious nerve signals constantly passes to and fro between muscles, spinal cord and brain, controlling these actions. It would take a high-speed computer to mimic the signals taking place in, for example, a skier.

The tendons play no active part in producing movements. They merely transmit the pull of their muscles through firm connections to bones. The Achilles tendon in this way transmits the pull of the calf muscles to the heel-bone. Joints, too, act passively, but they are vital for every movement. The shape of the joint,

whether it resembles a straight hinge, as in the elbow or knee, or is like a ball and socket, as in the hip, determines the type of movement possible. Pads of smooth, tough cartilage cover the bone ends, reducing friction and cushioning shock. The joint is lubricated by slippery synovial fluid which is contained in the capsule that encloses the joint.

Holding the two bones of a joint firmly together are tough but flexible ligaments. Some people have ligaments that are slacker than normal, resulting in hypermobility, or "double joints," which are not in fact double at all. One result of the right type of prolonged regular exercise is to increase the flexibility of joints by slightly stretching the ligaments. This is most commonly found in ballet dancers. Probably just as important in normal exercise, however, is simple "training" of the body to tolerate greater joint movement. Nerve signals fed back from the joints to the brain prevent joints from moving too far. This is an inborn protective measure, and exercise adapts the joints to greater movement. A hazard of many sports, however, is that certain joints are stretched too far, resulting in torn ligaments known as sprains, or even dislocations. Soccer players' knee ligaments are notoriously prone to injury.

But muscles are the basic seat of action. How is the muscular power generated that can lift a massive weight or produce the gentlest touch? As in every bodily process, the energy for muscular effort comes ultimately from food and involves a whole complex train of chemical reactions. These break down the chemical molecules of food, extracting the energy which holds them together.

The two food supplies most readily available to muscular tissues are glucose, a form of sugar that circulates dissolved in the blood, and glycogen, or animal starch, which is stored in the muscles themselves. The body has other food stores, but these are slower to mobilize and not much use in meeting immediate needs during exercise. They are the deposits of fat, mainly under the skin, and a store of glycogen in the liver which is partly converted into blood glucose by the hormone adrenaline released by the adrenal glands in response to stress. But fat deposits can be used only very slowly for supplying energy. What is more, a small amount of fat contains a large amount of food energy. It is for these reasons that exercise alone—without controlling your diet—is not an effective way of slimming.

The chemical reactions that break down such foods as glucose and glycogen normally need a constant supply of

You Exercise?

oxygen, the gas we breathe in from the air through our lungs. Oxygen is carried from the lungs by the red cells of the blood, and this in turn is pumped by the heart. The breakdown of foods produces two main waste products—water and the gas carbon dioxide. These, too, are carried away by the blood. The carbon dioxide is breathed out through the lungs, while the water is excreted in sweat and urine.

A constant blood supply and adequate breathing are of vital importance to effective muscular action and these must be increased during all forms of exercise.

The body has a sensitive built-in mechanism that adjusts breathing and heartbeat to meet the body's varying demands. There are, for example, receptors in the aorta, the main blood vessel leaving the heart, and the carotid artery, which supplies the brain, that react to any drop in the amount of oxygen in the blood. They send nerve signals to the heart, via the brain, increasing both the rate of its beat and the amount of blood pumped with each beat. In this way, the heart's output may be boosted from the normal five litres per minute at rest to more than 20 litres per minute during such vigorous exercises as a 100-yard swim.

In a similar way, the amount of air passing in and out of the lungs is greatly increased, by increasing both the depth of breathing and its rate. In this case, control is exerted by a part of the brain called the respiratory centre, which is sensitive to any rise in the amount of carbon dioxide dissolved in the blood. Other mechanisms also boost the supply to the muscles. The very act of muscular contraction, for example, helps to pump the blood back to the heart for recirculation around the body.

Although these reactions occur quite quickly, they are not instantaneous. It is when they have come fully into play, reaching peak efficiency, that an athlete experiences his "second wind." In some cases, however, a person deliberately forces his muscles to expend energy too quickly for the normal breakdown of food by oxygen to be able to keep up with the muscle tissues' needs. This happens, for example, during a sprint race, or if you do 20 press-ups in quick succession. Then an entirely different chain of chemical reactions can take place, allowing some, but not all, of the energy stored in food molecules to be released quickly without using oxygen.

The end product of these reactions is a substance called lactic acid, which collects in the muscles and causes an immediate feeling of fatigue. The only way to get rid of the lactic acid is to retrace the chemical pathway that produced it. This in itself requires energy and, therefore, oxygen. Following the lactic acid route incurs an "oxygen debt" that has to be repaid later. Hence the panting and racing heartbeat that follows for some time after a strenuous burst of activity.

Fatigue felt after a sprint is quite different from the muscular stiffness that follows unaccustomed physical effort. Apart from actual muscle strain, a major cause of this stiffness is oedema, a build-up of fluid in the muscle tissues. Stiffness may result if the water, which is a by-product of energy production in the muscles, is not carried away efficiently. In an unfit person, the muscles' blood vessels may not act efficiently, and muscle oedema may also be aggravated by raised blood pressure and by not "warming down" after exercise. It is a feeling which a person who is out of condition and plays tennis for several hours knows only too well. By continuing with gentle exercise for a short period of time after strenuous exertion, the draining of blood from the muscles can be aided. Stiffness can be reduced by massage or a hot bath. But adequate exercise resulting in physical fitness greatly reduces this complaint.

One of the reasons for this, and a major reason for undergoing any programme of exercises, is that training increases the efficiency of the entire cardio-vascular (heart and blood vessel)

Just when exercise becomes unbearable, when you're out of breath and your muscles ache, you find new energy. What is "second wind"?

and respiratory (breathing) systems. The heart is built principally of a special type of muscular tissue and the pumping action of breathing is also muscular. And exercise of any muscle results in hypertrophy, or an increase in size and strength, provided that the diet contains enough protein to build the new tissues. On the other hand giving up an exercise programme reduces muscle strength again and total lack of use results in atrophy. Thus exercise strengthens both the muscles actually being used, and because it indirectly exercises the heart and breathing muscles, exercise also increases heart-lung power.

In neither case, however, is it much use doing mild exercises that need little effort. Exercise only strengthens any muscle if the majority of its fibres are

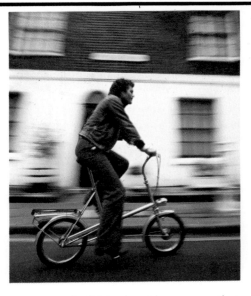

being used. This is the reason that exercising with one-pound weights is no use in strengthening the arms. Thus effective exercise, whether it be running, swimming, an exercise programme or some form of sport, should make a person comfortably tired and out of breath, perhaps doubling the heart rate from its normal figure of more than 70 beats per minute. This does no harm to a healthy person. It is the body's normal way of meeting increased needs. However, anyone who has had a heart attack or who has heart trouble should always follow his doctor's advice regarding exercise.

As the result of regular exercise for a sufficient period of time, the heart's muscle fibres become stronger and its chambers larger than before. Fewer strokes are needed to move the same amount of blood, and the heart rate will be slower both at rest and at a particular level of exercise. Moreover, the maximum output—which is reached in both trained and untrained hearts at a rate of about 180 beats per minute—is greatly increased. These effects are seen most dramatically in Olympic athletes, whose hearts beat much more slowly than the average person's. But anyone can achieve a worthwhile improvement through physical training.

Much the same thing happens with breathing as the chest muscles become stronger and the amount of air which can be breathed in and out of the lungs increases. One of the most noticeable effects of regular exercise is that the drop to a normal pulse and breathing rate occurs more quickly. This is the simple result of increased heart-lung efficiency, so that levels of oxygen and waste products in the body return to normal more rapidly.

One "waste product" of physical exertion is heat. Any mechanical system that is not 100 per cent efficient—and none are—produces waste heat, and the body is no exception. Muscular effort greatly increases heat output. This excess must be discarded, for the body works most efficiently at its "normal" temperature of 37 °C (98.6 °F). Very sensitive centres in the brain detect any change in the core temperature, that of the blood and internal organs, and bring compensating mechanisms into action. In particular, the flow of blood to the skin is increased and so is sweating. Evaporation of the sweat carries away much excess heat.

If these mechanisms break down, when a person undertakes too much exercise in excessive temperatures, perhaps, the result is heat-stroke. Another hazard of prolonged exertion leading to excessive sweating is the well-known loss of salt, resulting in cramp. This is the reason that marathon runners, miners and others who exert themselves over long periods must take salt tablets. However, this is not likely to trouble the ordinary person, and a much more common cause of cramp in non-athletes is simple over-exertion of untrained muscles. This can be prevented by developing any exercise programme slowly and steadily.

Ironically, warming-up before a bout of physical activity seems not to increase the temperature of the body. While muscle temperature may rise slightly, and there is, perhaps, a feeling of warmth due to the flow of extra blood to the skin, experiments show that limbering up is not enough to raise the core temperature. In fact, there is some controversy as to what, if anything, warming-up does achieve, beyond psychological preparedness for an athletic event.

There are, however, two main possibilities. First, warming-up may "prime" the circulatory system, increasing its output so that it can more easily respond to the increased demands to come. Second, it may renew the body's adaptation to the nervous mechanism that normally guards the joints, preventing excessive movement. In other words, "loosening-up" does not physically make the body's joints looser, but it does accustom them to undergoing greater movements than normal. And that is just as important for the man or woman who uses simple exercise routines to keep his or her body in trim as it is for the international athlete who is trying to beat an Olympic record.

Sports medicine and physiology is a relatively young field, but its benefits spread far from the sports arena. Because an efficiently functioning body is vital for survival and a proper programme of exercise increases bodily efficiency, every individual can benefit from a knowledge of how the body functions when undergoing exercise. It is not necessary to be an expert physiologist, but when you understand how and why various parts of your body react as they do it will be easier for you to adapt any form of exercise to your individual needs. This is the case if you favour swimming or golf, walking or calesthenics. The basic principles are always the same.

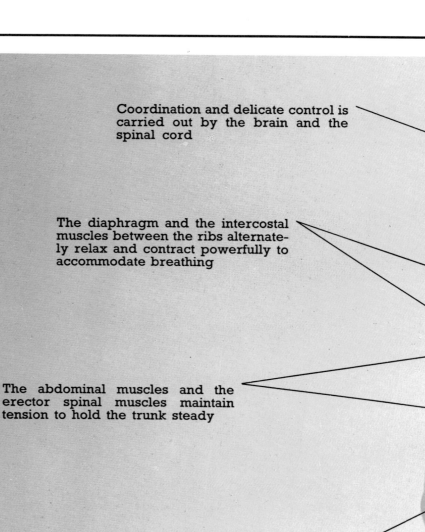

Coordination and delicate control is carried out by the brain and the spinal cord

The diaphragm and the intercostal muscles between the ribs alternately relax and contract powerfully to accommodate breathing

The abdominal muscles and the erector spinal muscles maintain tension to hold the trunk steady

The quadriceps at the front of the thigh and the hamstring group at the back of the thighs act alternately to flex and straighten the legs, aided by the gluteal muscles of the buttocks

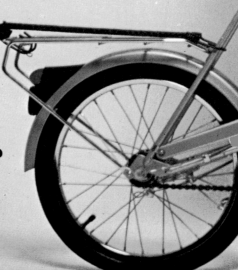

What Happens When You Exercise?

No matter what form of exercise you take, the effects on the body are basically the same—your heart rate increases, your joints move, your muscles contract and lengthen. This diagram illustrates what happens to your body when you ride a bicycle.

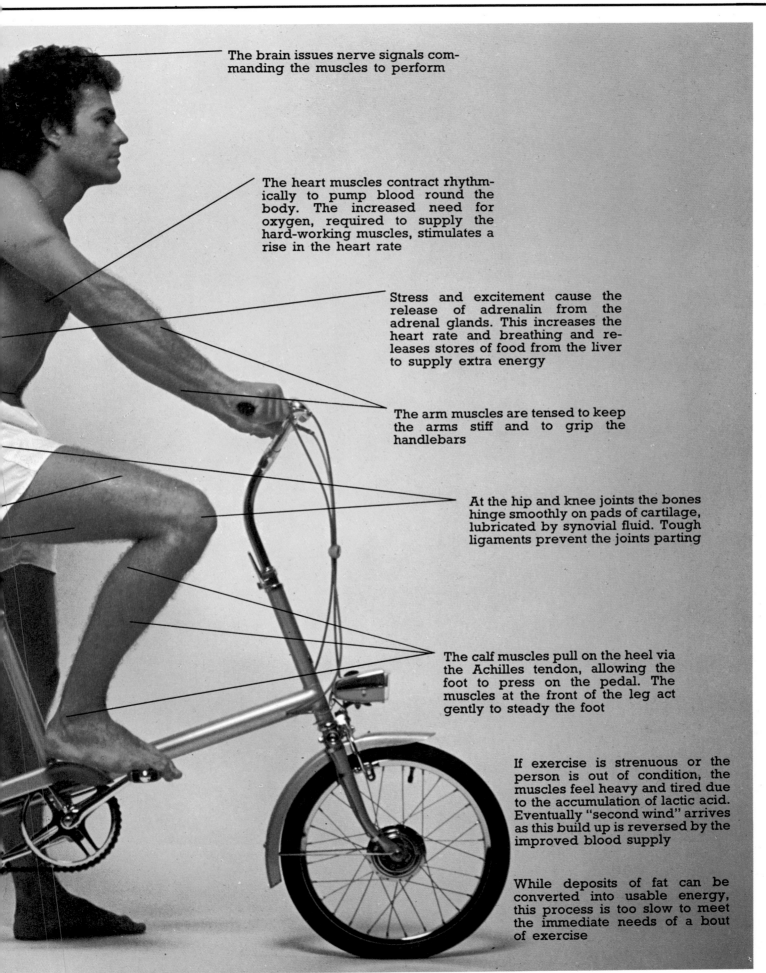

The brain issues nerve signals commanding the muscles to perform

The heart muscles contract rhythmically to pump blood round the body. The increased need for oxygen, required to supply the hard-working muscles, stimulates a rise in the heart rate

Stress and excitement cause the release of adrenalin from the adrenal glands. This increases the heart rate and breathing and releases stores of food from the liver to supply extra energy

The arm muscles are tensed to keep the arms stiff and to grip the handlebars

At the hip and knee joints the bones hinge smoothly on pads of cartilage, lubricated by synovial fluid. Tough ligaments prevent the joints parting

The calf muscles pull on the heel via the Achilles tendon, allowing the foot to press on the pedal. The muscles at the front of the leg act gently to steady the foot

If exercise is strenuous or the person is out of condition, the muscles feel heavy and tired due to the accumulation of lactic acid. Eventually "second wind" arrives as this build up is reversed by the improved blood supply

While deposits of fat can be converted into usable energy, this process is too slow to meet the immediate needs of a bout of exercise

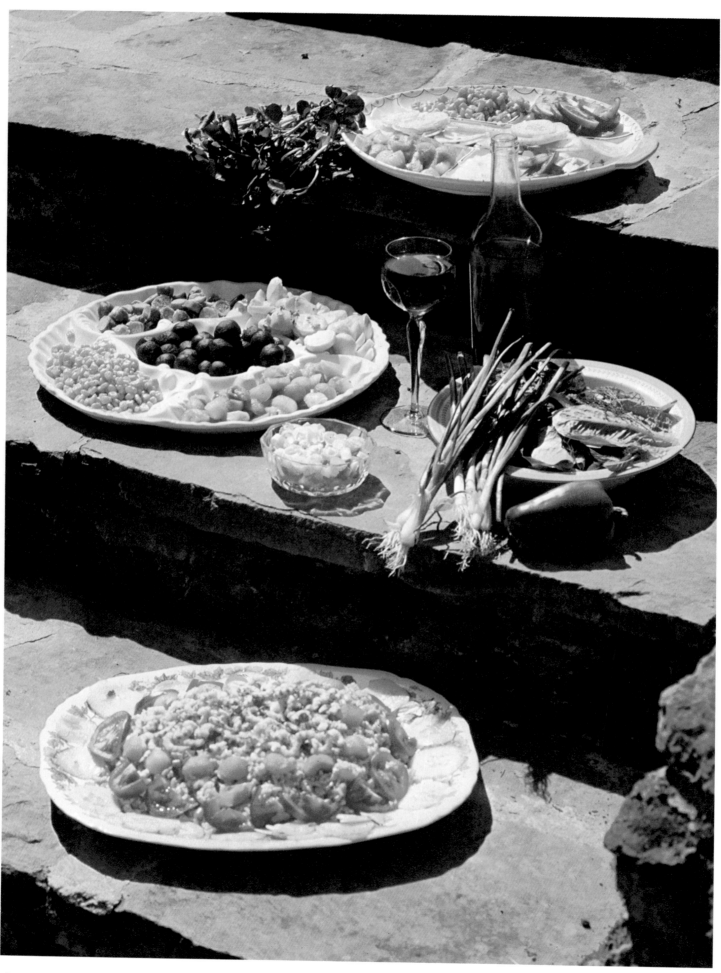

Eating for Energy

To feel well and to enjoy life we really need to have plenty of energy and vitality. We need energy for all the different kinds of physical activity that work and an active social life demand. We also need energy to carry out the semi-automatic life processes of basal metabolism which are essential to keep us alive. We need energy to build new tissues, to keep existing ones in good repair and working as efficiently as possible. We need energy to think, for our nerves to pass impulses around our bodies and to keep ourselves warm.

The body's primary nutritional requirement is for energy. This need will be satisfied above all others. Although, for example, the main function of protein is the maintenance of body tissues, if the energy intake from carbohydrate foods falls short of the body's requirement, protein will be broken down only for energy. This may be to the detriment of the tissues which need constant renewal of damaged cells.

If the energy intake is reduced for any length of time, the body's fat stores are mobilized to make good the energy deficit. This is what happens, of course, on a weight-reducing diet when you simply use up your stored energy instead of getting an equivalent amount of energy from your food. If, for one reason or another, the energy intake drops to a very low level, after the fat

Energy! Vitality! Vigour! Why be satisfied with anything less? You can learn how to eat for energy and enjoy life to the fullest.

stores have been depleted, the protein in the body tissues themselves may be broken down for energy.

Carbohydrates, fats and proteins can all be used by the body as sources of energy. These nutrients are broken down inside the body's cells and the energy stored within the molecules of each nutrient is liberated. This energy is

then made available for the body's use.

The energy-release process is actually a continuous chain of chemical reactions. Chemical tools, called enzymes, help to split up the molecules to release the energy. For these chemical reactions to proceed efficiently, a regular supply of some of the B-group vitamins is required. Vitamin B_1, or thiamine, Vitamin B_2, or riboflavin, and niacin act as enzyme assistants, co-enzymes, to start off the chain of reactions and to regulate the whole process.

As enzyme assistants, the B vitamins are rather like the tool which holds the nut as the screwdriver—which is analogous to the enzyme—turns the bolt, where the nut and bolt together represent the nutrient molecule to be broken down. So although carbohydrate, in the form of either starch or sugar, and fats and proteins are necessary to provide a source of energy, these B vitamins are essential for the release of this energy.

The whole range of B vitamins will be supplied by a varied and well-balanced

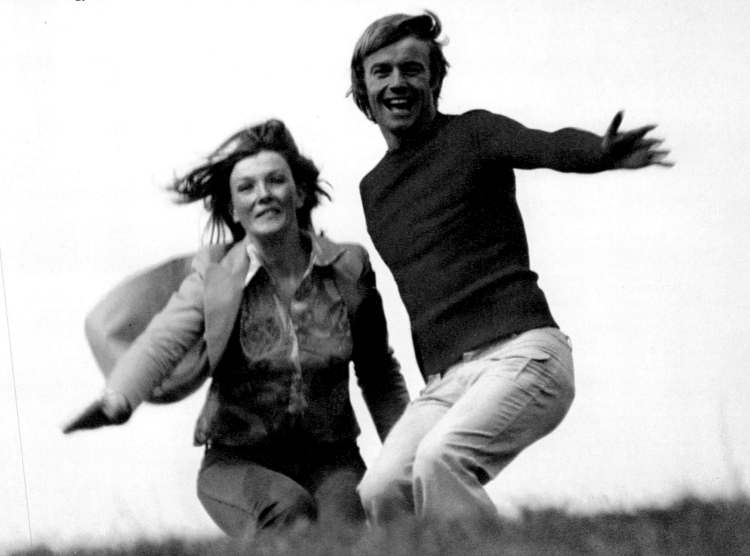

diet. The richest sources of the B vitamins are all kinds of meat, especially pork, liver, kidney and heart, wholemeal and enriched white flours—and therefore foods like bread which are made from flour—eggs, dairy produce and such vegetables as peas and beans.

In addition to the nutrients which yield the energy, and a good supply of the B vitamins to assist in its release, you also need oxygen because energy is liberated in a process called oxidation. Oxygen is carried in the blood to every cell in the body. The oxygen diffuses through the thin walls of the lungs into the tiny blood vessels which form a fine network around the lungs. There the oxygen latches on to the red pigment—haemoglobin—of the red blood cells. Then as oxyhaemoglobin it is carried around to every cell in the body. When blood flows past cells which require more oxygen, this detaches itself from the haemoglobin, and enters the cell to play its part in the cellular reactions.

It is clear that to provide a good supply of oxygen to the cells, the blood needs its full quota of haemoglobin. Like all the other tissues of the body, the basic constituents of haemoglobin—iron and protein—come from a balanced diet.

Many people, especially women, who feel lethargic, perpetually weary or find that the slightest exertion leaves them exhausted may be suffering from iron-deficiency anaemia. This is remarkably common even in countries where the diet is generally good. In Great Britain it is estimated that about one-tenth of the adult female population suffers from this type of anaemia. The United States Department of Agriculture, too, reports an alarmingly high incidence of anaemia.

Anaemia of this kind is caused by a shortage of iron in the body, which in turn may be the long-term result of a deficient diet, or of massive or regular blood loss. Women are particularly prone to anaemia because of menstruation.

On the whole, while iron in animal food sources is more available to the body than that in vegetable sources, only about 10 per cent of the iron in the food you eat is available for absorption into the body. Vitamin C assists in the absorption of this iron.

Once iron is absorbed into the body, however, it is lost only very slowly. The average life span of a red blood cell is 120 days. It is then broken down and the iron is recycled in the formation of new red blood cells.

When there is a shortage of iron, the body replaces worn-out blood cells with new ones which are low in haemoglobin. This means that the blood cannot carry its normal load of oxygen. And this in turn limits the rate at which food can be broken down to supply energy. The most practical solution to iron-deficiency anaemia is a course of iron tablets prescribed by a doctor.

But prevention is always better than cure, and it is vital to include iron-rich foods among the general groups of food for energy. By a fortunate coincidence, many of the most important dietary sources of the B vitamins also contain more iron than other foods. So, to avoid becoming anaemic, it is a good idea to eat plenty of meat—especially liver, kidney and heart—wholemeal cereals and enriched white flours, eggs and vegetables.

Finally, for the reaction between food material and oxygen to occur, two other vitamins are needed. Although their precise role is not yet understood, it is known that both vitamin C and vitamin E are essential for metabolic processes. Vitamin C is found in many fruits and vegetables, but the citrus fruits—oranges, lemons, grapefruit—berries or summer fruits—blackcurrants and strawberries—and green vegetables are the best sources. Vitamin E is widespread in many different kinds of food. Fats and oils, vegetables and cereal foods supply most of the vitamin E in our diets.

It would be very nice to think that the more of the energy foods you eat, the more energetic and dynamic you become. But the body breaks down only enough food to meet its present energy demand. The long-term result of eating too much food is, in the vast majority of cases, to put the excess energy into storage as fat. And the usual consequence is an increase in weight, not energy.

Many nutritionists advise that, for moderately active people, 15 per cent of the day's energy be supplied by proteins from meat, fish, cheese, milk and eggs, that about 35 per cent of the daily energy requirement comes from such fats as butter and margarine, as well as the so-called "invisible" fats in such foods as milk, cheese, eggs and nuts. The remaining 50 per cent should come from carbohydrates—from the starch of bread, potatoes, pasta, rice and other cereal foods and from the sugar in vegetables and fresh and dried fruits. With these proportions, the diet is usually a nutritionally well-balanced one. It should also satisfy any need for other important nutrients such as proteins and vitamins. Such a diet should prove to be quite a palatable one, too, which is neither monotonous nor starchy.

It is obvious that the more energetic an individual is the more energy his daily food must supply. Many people, for example, who spend five days a week sitting at a desk find that they eat more at weekends when they are more physically active. The working wife who catches up with her housework on Saturday, and her husband who plays a game of football or a round of golf will have bigger appetites on Saturday and Sunday than they have during the week.

It is easy to understand this, but nutritionists are still searching for the physiological reasons why people who are the same age, weight and sex, and lead equally active lives can vary so

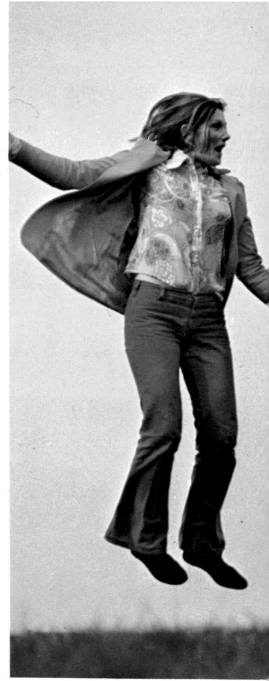

much in the amount of energy foods they require. Taking the population as a whole, it is possible to find one person who needs four times as much food as another, although both of them seem to use up the same amount of energy. This does explain, of course, why one person can eat enormously and stay thin while another person eats much less, but puts on weight easily. In discussing energy requirements, average values must be used, but it is necessary to bear in mind that variations are considerable.

Just as energy requirements vary from person to person, they also vary throughout life. Related to body weight, energy requirements gradually fall from birth onwards. In relation to his body weight the infant has the greatest energy requirement. The growing child needs

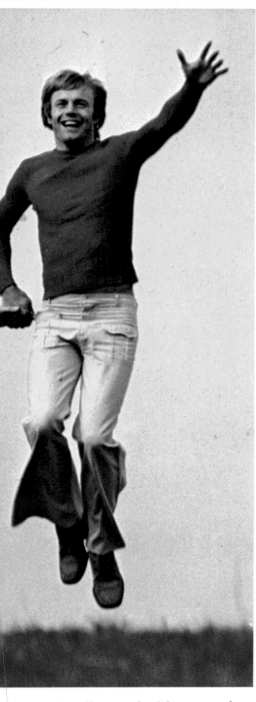

daily energy requirement may reach 2,500 Calories. During pregnancy the metabolic rate—or the rate at which energy is used in the body—speeds up. This is due to the rapid growth and development of the foetus in addition to the gradual building up of maternal tissues. On the other hand, in the West most women tend to become less active as their pregnancy advances. The increased metabolism and the decreased activity may balance one another out. In this case, the expectant mother does not need to increase the overall energy value of the food she eats. Often her diet needs careful management to ensure that her increased protein, mineral and vitamin requirements are met without exceeding the energy level she requires.

Most men need enough food to give them about 2,700 Calories a day, 3,000 if they are fairly active, and up to 3,600 if they lead very active lives. In the past men doing such heavy manual work as mining, forestry or farming might have needed up to 5,000 Calories a day. Due to increased modern mechanization, these very high levels of activity are now rarely encountered. If they are, they are not maintained for long periods. But athletes, when they are in strict training, may need up to 5,000 Calories a day because they will "burn up" this amount of food during sustained physical activity.

Although energy requirements may be well above average, extra activity does not increase the body's need for proteins, minerals and vitamins, apart from certain B-group vitamins. Since these vitamins are concerned with energy release a good supply is necessary in a high energy diet. Theoretically, the greater energy needs could be met by eating extra large helpings of the major carbohydrate foods, such as bread, potatoes and pasta. But a diet in which more than half the energy comes exclusively from carbohydrate tends to be dull and too starchy. It is best to eat more of all kinds of foods so that the proportions of the overall energy requirement derived from protein, fats and carbohydrates will remain at 15 per cent, 35 per cent and 50 per cent respectively.

Most people become less active as they grow older. Although there are some people just as active at 70 years old as they were at 50 or even 30 years old, they are in the minority. For everyone, basal metabolism slows down with increasing age, and so we all need to eat less food for energy as we get older.

Usually an elderly person's energy requirement is best met by reducing the number of calories derived from carbohydrate. When total energy requirements are low, they must be met by those foods which satisfy the body's other nutritional requirements as well. For example, to have enough protein in her diet, an elderly woman may need to eat a daily portion of meat, half a pint of milk, one ounce of cheese, an egg and three ounces of bread. These foods would also supply

her with 900 Calories or almost half her total energy requirement. The rest should be supplied by fruit and vegetables. When energy requirements are low, there is certainly no place in the diet for "empty" calories.

Everyone knows the feeling of fatigue associated with hunger. Whatever a person's overall energy requirements, there are often times during the day when he feels drained of energy. Yet with even a small meal, you suddenly feel much brighter. Normally, a certain amount of sugar—blood sugar—derived from the normal digestion of food is carried in the blood stream. Usually the blood-sugar level is kept steady by additional energy reserves of glycogen in the liver.

In times of stress or in an emergency you may need to be able to act very swiftly. Under these conditions, increased quantities of adrenaline circulating in the blood mobilize glycogen from the liver which causes a rapid rise in the level of blood sugar. This extra supply of fuel is used to meet the increased demands for energy.

Three or four hours after a meal these glycogen reserves are used up and, consequently, the level of blood sugar drops. This lowered level is thought to be one of the mechanisms which stimulates the appetite. But if you don't eat in response to these signals, you might feel tired and become light-headed. If you eat a meal, the blood-sugar level is quickly re-established.

Obviously there is a time lag between eating and feeling more energetic, although food can give an immediate psychological lift. During this time lag, the food has to be digested before it can enter the blood stream and boost the flagging blood-sugar level. For this reason, foods that are quickly digested have a more rapid effect. Sugar is digested more quickly than starch, which in turn is digested more quickly than protein and far more quickly than fats. Fats and fatty foods stay much longer in the stomach than other foods. This is why foods with a high fat content keep hunger pangs at bay, whereas a meal that is mainly carbohydrate is quickly digested.

A well-balanced meal with plenty of proteins and some fats is the most sustaining of all. There will be a rapid rise in the level of blood sugar as the carbohydrates are digested. Then this blood-sugar level will be kept up by the slower digestion of the protein and fats. Some people feel the effects of low blood sugar more acutely than others. While some can go for many hours without food and feel none the worse for it, others need the "little and often" kind of meal pattern if they are to feel at their energetic best all day long.

By experimentation, by eating a widely varied diet, by seeing how you feel when you eat three meals a day or four or five smaller meals you can determine what and how you can best eat for energy.

proportionally more food for energy than an adult does. This is because the actual growing process, which is really the building of new body cells, creates a great demand for energy. For both boys and girls the period in life when energy requirements may reach their upper limit is during the great growth spurt of adolescence. Boys between the ages of 15 and 18 years will need up to 3,000 Calories a day, and perhaps even more than this if they are very active. Girls usually develop earlier than boys, so their period of maximum growth can be anywhere from nine to 18 years of age, when they need about 2,300 Calories.

Still using average values, most women between the ages of 18 and 55 will need enough food to supply 2,200 Calories each day. If she is very active, a woman's

THE PRINCIPAL VITAMINS

Common name	Chemical name(s)	Good sources	Daily needs	What it does for you	Discovery date
A	Retinol	Fish liver oils, animal liver, eggs, milk, yogurt, butter, green leafy vegetables, carrots.	2.7 mg	Essential for body growth and proper function of the retina. Helps resistance to infections.	1913
B1	Thiamine, aneurine	Yeast, wheat germ, wholemeal wholewheat flour, lean meat.	1.2 mg	Essential factor in carbohydrate metabolism. Important for nervous system, digestive system and heart. Severe lack causes beriberi which can lead to heart failure and damage to the nervous system.	1936
B2	Riboflavin	Yeast, wheat germ, liver, kidneys, cheese, meat.	1.7 mg	Important for normal growth of skin, nails and hair. Deficiency causes dull hair, split fingernails, itching eyes.	1933
B6	Pyridoxine	Yeast, wheat germ, liver, potatoes.	1.5 mg	For healthy skin and proper growth in children.	1936
	Niacin nicotinic acid,	Yeast, wheat, bread, liver, meat, fish, chicken, mushrooms.	19 mg	For healthy skin (anti-pellagra), mucous membranes and nervous system.	1937
(H)	Biotin	Yeast, peanuts, peas, mushrooms.	Unknown	Uncertain	1940
	Pantothenic acid	Yeast, liver, beans, mushrooms, peanuts.	Unknown	Uncertain	1938
	Folic acid	Yeast, liver, milk, green vegetables.	0.15 mg	Healthy blood	1944
B12	Cyanocobalamin	Liver, meat, wholemeal (wholewheat) flour, wheat germ.	0.005 mg	Healthy blood. This is known as the anti-pernicious anaemia vitamin.	1948
C	Ascorbic acid	Fresh fruit and vegetables especially citrus fruits, blackcurrants, tomatoes, rosehips.	30 mg	Vitality, resistance to infections, helps the body to resist shock, too. Essential for the formation of the body 'cement' which holds together the inter-cellular material making up the connective tissue, bones, teeth and blood-vessel walls.	1928
D	Calciferol	Fish liver oils, eggs, milk, butter, sunshine on skin.	0.01 mg	Regulates calcium and phosphorous content of the body. (This is essential in teeth and bone formation). Mostly needed during childhood but essential, too, during pregnancy.	1922
E	Tocopherol	Wheat germ, whole grains, nuts, vegetable oils.	Unknown	Protects body tissues. Keeps blood circulating freely.	1923
K		Green vegetables, liver, tomatoes, carrot tops, soya bean oil, seaweed.	Unknown	Essential for maintenance of prothrombin, one of the blood-clotting factors in blood plasma. Therefore helps to heal wounds.	1935

THE PRINCIPAL MINERALS

Common name	Chemical name	Good sources	What it does for you
Calcium	Ca	Milk, cheese, sardines or other small fish eaten whole with bones, parsley, watercress, molasses.	All body cells need calcium. Essential for the formation of bones, teeth, hair, fingernails. Protects the nervous system, helps blood clotting and is important in maintaining healthy body fluids, membrane and muscles. Particularly vital for growing children and pregnant women. (Calcium needs vitamin D to aid absorption).
Cobalt	Co	Sweetbreads, mushrooms, liver.	Constituent of vitamin B12 and concerned with the promotion of healthy nerve fibres and tissues of the bone Guards against types of anaemia.
Copper	Cu	Liver, kidney, egg yolk, lentils, wholemeal (wholewheat) flour, parsley, brown sugar, brazil nuts and walnuts.	Concerned with several enzyme systems including those responsible for the oxidation of vitamin C.
Fluorine	F	Drinking water in certain areas, seafoods, tea (particularly China tea).	Builds up tooth enamel in children and guards against tooth decay.
Iodine	I	Seafoods, Kelp, sea salt. Fruit, vegetables and cereals may contain supplies but amounts vary depending on area.	Essential for correct functioning of the thyroid gland, guards against goitre, keeps body cells and circulation active. Also assists in healthy development of the brain and continuing sexual interest.
Iron	Fe	Egg yolk, liver, black pudding (blood sausage), molasses, corned beef, peanuts, lentils and some green vegetables (e.g. watercress).	Helps make blood. During child-bearing years women need more iron than men (they lose large amounts during menstruation). Iron is also concerned with the formation of body cells and production of energy. Deficiency may cause anaemia.
Magnesium	Mg	Green salads, green vegetables, nuts, beans, lentils, whole grains.	Concerned with strength and well-being of bones, teeth, nerves, muscles, hair and nails.
Manganese	Mn	Liver, kidney, beans, lentils, cereals, tea and coffee, nuts.	Activator in a number of enzyme systems. A deficiency in animals produces poor growth and reproduction, and occasional anaemia. It can also cause bone changes and disturbances in the central nervous system and a disappearance of sexual drive.
Phosphorus	P	Milk, cheese, egg yolk, yeast, wholemeal (wholewheat) flour, nuts, meat.	Helps make bones, teeth, body cells and tissues, hair and fingernails. Helps the release of energy during the processing of carbohydrates. Phosphorus needs vitamin D to assist absorption. Many of the B group of vitamins work only when combined with phosphates in the body.
Potassium	K	Dried apricots, beans, nuts, dried currants, dates, figs, grapes, prunes, raisins, sultanas, soya flour, molasses, yeast, brown sugar.	Works with sodium to maintain a correct fluid balance. Essential for heart rhythm, nerve activity and the processing of carbohydrates.
Selenium	Se	Liver, kidney, heart.	Acts with vitamin E to maintain a healthy condition of the liver and also to inhibit the development of muscular dystrophy.
Sodium	Na	Dried apricots, beans, nuts, table salt, ham, bread, beef extract, celery, eggs, spinach,	Acts with potassium to correct fluid balance.
Sulphur	S	Nuts, dried fruits, oatmeal, barley, beans, cheese, meat,	Helps in the construction and maintenance of body cells and muscle fibres.
Zinc	Z	Oysters, sweetbreads, liver.	Involved in several enzyme systems and constituent of insulin. Eyes, teeth and testes all contain considerable amounts.

Check your posture

Are you sitting comfortably? And what is even more important, are you sitting correctly?

Stand up and take a quick look at yourself in a mirror. Do your shoulders look hunched? Does your stomach or bottom stick out? Are your feet pointing outwards in penguin fashion? After that glimpse of yourself are you automatically straightening up and trying to improve your posture? Don't, that would only be pretending. What you want to find out is how you hold yourself when you are not suddenly made self-conscious about it. The test is how your posture rates when no one is looking.

Bad posture, like long hair, has the reputation of being a peculiarity of the young. Members of the older generation tend to say that in their day, they had to sit up straight at school, stand up straight in the army—and that young people today slouch about all over the place. Although it is certainly true that many young people *do* stand and sit badly—the same is *also* true of older people. When their guard is down they relax into bad habits.

Why it's important to hold yourself well

It's not simply a question of looking good —although anyone can look better if they do stand well—there are definite health reasons. The way you sit or stand vitally affects your physical structure as it does your appearance and personality.

Put your back into it!

The backbone is the 'kingpin' of the body's skeletal system. It forms a solid but flexible upright structure which gives support to the rest of the body while remaining supple itself. It is a very neat piece of 'engineering'—consisting of no less than 33 small bones, with slightly moveable joints between so that the bones can twist and slide against each other.

The backbone isn't quite straight. It forms an elongated 'S' shape, curving very slightly from the neck to the chest, back slightly towards the waist region then forward again to the hip region where nine bones are joined together to form a rigid support for the hip girdle. Inevitably, bad posture will strain this complicated mechanism.

But don't get the impression that your backbone is too delicate to allow you to *use* it. Instead, enjoy back-bending activities like gardening, or games involving bending—and counteract the effect by employing good posture at all times. Simple posture exercises will help to ease tension and keep your backbone supple.

Follow the exercise programme

Has the check list convinced you? If going through our check-list has made you sit up, then start to think about doing something *positive* to improve your posture. It is not enough to stand up straight now and then when your conscience pricks, then slump back into a heap again. What is needed is a good sitting and standing pose which becomes automatic—and you will almost certainly need to eradicate posture *faults* before this can be achieved.

Because good posture is usually a relatively simple thing to achieve, this is one area of physical well-being where *you* can take control. Don't be too disheartened if you don't score very highly in the Mirror Test. Even models have to be taught how to stand, walk and sit correctly. At first you may feel a little self-conscious about remembering to stand up straight and pull your shoulders back. You may think your posture is slightly exaggerated. It won't be. So keep at it until you develop a natural stance which is easy on the eye and you'll find it much more comfortable too.

Good posture can be used in simple everyday situations like checking a shoestrap, lifting and carrying, reading and writing. If you have heavy parcels to carry then make sure the weight is evenly distributed and walk tall—don't stoop. You'll look graceful and poised and you'll avoid the tension which leads to backache and other associated problems.

The next chapter gives you a complete programme of exercises designed to improve posture. We take you through the simplest bodily positions from how to sit at work or at play, the kind of chairs to choose to keep you sitting comfortably and correctly, to the way to stand whether you are holding still or walking. You can try them out and you'll notice the improvement immediately. You may find that those figure problems are simply the result of years of bad posture!

Posture, balance and co-ordination

Children instinctively appreciate the value of good co-ordination and proper balance. You can see it in their games. They walk quickly without stepping on lines in the pavement, and skip with the rope swung at alternating speeds. If these games were continued beyond childhood, if this sort of training became part of our daily lives, there would be more champion swimmers and graceful dancers, more poise, grace and elegance in evidence than there is today.

Balance and co-ordination are intimately related. In many ways, they describe the same phenomenon. Internally, the body functions in a remarkably balanced and co-ordinated fashion, with the muscles, organs and hormones performing automatically to fulfil the synchronized requirements of living.

Externally, it's something else. Some people are naturally well co-ordinated and come equipped, even in childhood, with an excellent sense of balance. Without half-trying, they can perform two tasks simultaneously, dialling a telephone number, for example, while poking about for a fallen pencil just barely within reach. They can sit on high ledges without the slightest concern about the danger of falling off.

Good co-ordination and a sense of balance are often inherited. However, although the balance-control mechanism in the brain is more efficient in some people than in others, anybody can train to give greater bodily equilibrium and to co-ordinate movements more effectively.

One of the unsung heroines of history is the first teacher who put a book on top of a little girl's head and made her walk across the room without either touching or dropping it. The purpose was to improve the girl's posture. But what it did for her balance at the same time was just as important.

Good posture is more than just attractive. It is crucial to both co-ordination and balance. Good posture provides a focus for both, giving the body a stable, reliable centre of gravity from which to take its bearings. The ultimate reward is not just in bodily performance. A person who moves awkwardly wastes an enormous amount of effort, while someone whose body operates harmoniously will have plenty of energy left over at the end of the day for pleasure and recreation.

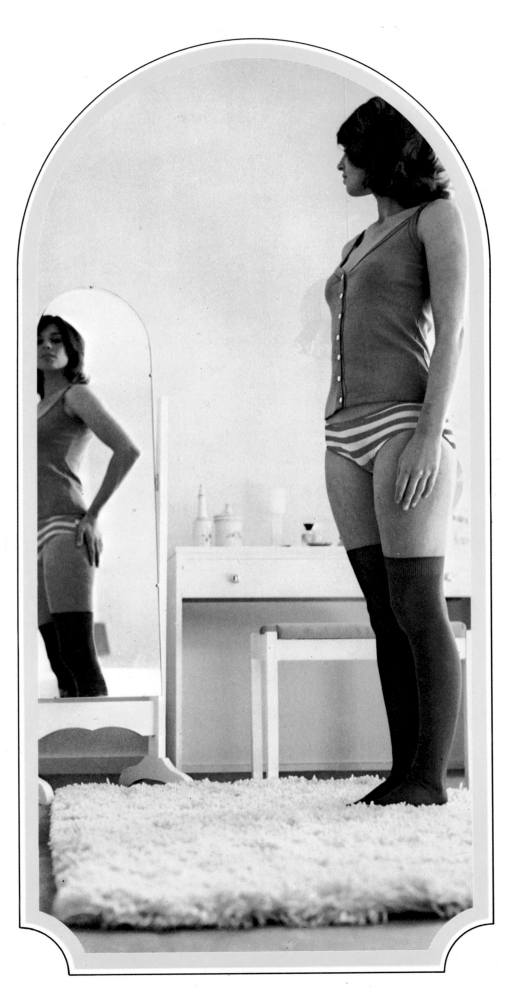

The mirror test

Try this easy check routine to find out just how harmful the effects of bad posture can be for you.

If the **head** is allowed to poke forward, shoulders hunched in a 'Dowager's Hump', then the mass of vital muscles and nerves at the base of the neck will become strained, leading to tiredness, backache, and possibly even arthritis in later years.

If the **shoulders** sag forward, then the chest will be cramped and the lungs will not be able to expand fully. If insufficient oxygen is taken in, then the body cells which depend on oxygen will not get their fair share, and you will feel tired and be less resistant to disease.

If the **backbone** is not held upright, then the digestive system, stomach and intestines will be cramped. Food will not be able to move along the intestines properly or be properly 'processed' in the stomach. Heartburn, indigestion, constipation and other stomach troubles could result.

If the **hip girdle** tilts forward or backwards or sideways, and the backbone is crooked too, then hump back, hollow waist or other deformities can develop. This is particularly true for growing children whose bones are still developing. The organs within the body's bone structure could be permanently cramped —leading to improper breathing, digestion, circulation and other ailments.

If the whole **body** sags, then muscles have to work harder to keep you upright at all. The ones that have to take the extra strain will naturally become tired. And so will you.

If the **feet** are not used properly, then the muscles will not contract and relax in the correct sequence, and the circulation will be slowed down. This can lead to night cramp and aching feet, as well as chillblains in winter.

Take a good critical look at yourself in the mirror and check the following points to find out how your posture rates. Here's the kind of thing you should be aiming for:

Head held up
Shoulders relaxed and back
Chest out
Back held straight but not stiff
Stomach muscles held firm
Bottom pulled in
Hips held at the same level
Feet balancing weight easily and evenly

25

Exercises to improve posture

These special exercises will help correct your postural faults and give you a natural stance which is both attractive *and* good for your health. It's a simple routine to practise in your bedroom. Repeat them daily for one week to encourage the development of good posture. Subsequently, a weekly run-through will help ensure that you keep these good habits going. Use the exercises after any strenuous activity such as gardening, decorating, or polishing floors, to relax and also tone your spine, shoulders and back. You'll notice that the improved stance will make your figure look better immediately.

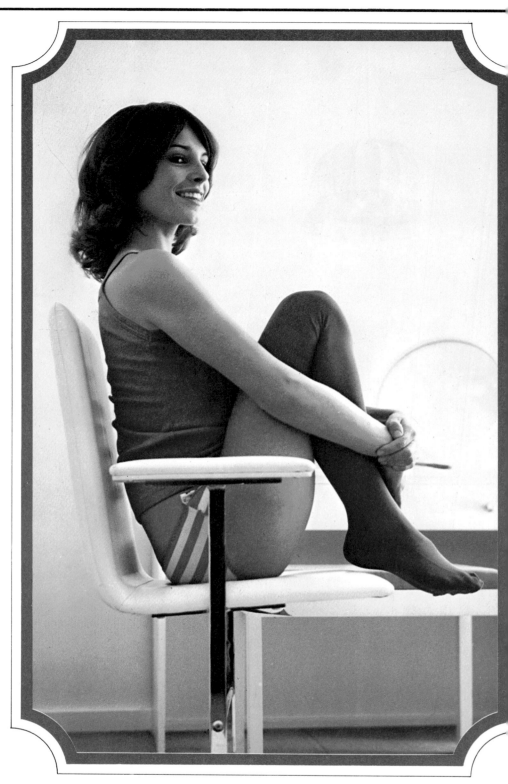

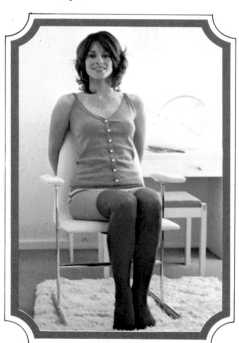

Exercise 1

Above Sit on a straight-backed chair, keep your back flat against the chair-back with your knees together and your feet flat on the floor. Now clasp your forearms behind the chair-back, bringing shoulders back as you do so. Hold for count of 10 and relax. Try to use a chair with a back that doesn't come above the middle of your back. Repeat three times.
Breathing Breathe regularly.

Exercise 2

Above Still sitting on a chair, with your bottom well back, and back straight. Raise your knees and pull them well in towards your chest, clasping them with your arms. Your feet must not touch the chair, and you must keep your back straight. Hold for a count of five, then lower slowly. Repeat three times.
Breathing Breathe in then out as you raise your knees.

Exercise 3

Below Sit on the edge of a stool or chair with your feet together and your knees bent. Now relax forward over your knees with head and arms down. Sweep your hands rhythmically forwards, backwards, forwards again and up then backwards. Follow the direction of your arms with your head. Repeat five times.
Breathing Breathe out as you relax over your knees and in as you stretch.

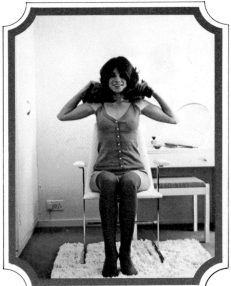

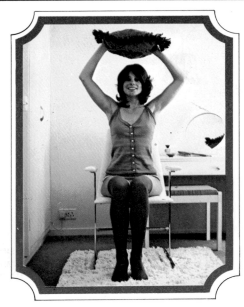

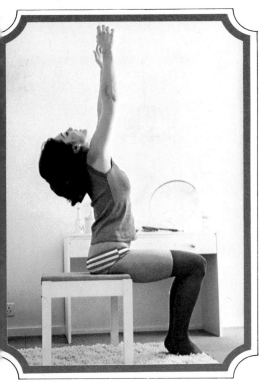

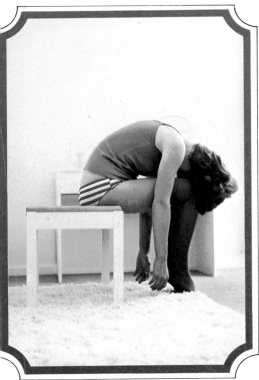

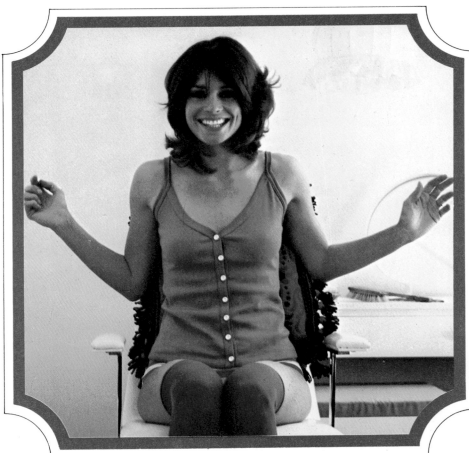

Exercise 4

Above Still in a sitting position, hold a cushion or pillow firmly on your knees. Your back should be about three inches away from the chair-back. Now raise your arms so that the cushion is above you, then lower them so that it rests just behind your neck. Hold for count of two. Now release the cushion and catch it between the lower part of your back and the chair-back. The movement should be rapid with a good backward movement of the lower part of your back. Repeat twice.
Breathing Breathe in as you raise the cushion, out as you lower it behind your back, then regularly as you release and catch it.

Exercise 5

Right Sit or stand with your back straight and head up. Now place a hard-back book on your head. Keeping your body completely still, turn your head to look over your left shoulder—without dropping the book. Return to the front position and repeat to the right. Repeat the whole movement four times.

Breathing Breathe regularly.

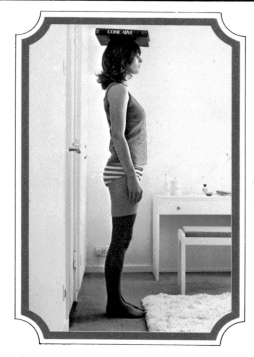

Exercise 6

Below Stand up straight in a doorway and place your hands behind your head, elbows well out. Your elbows should rest just inside the door frame. Now step very slightly through the door, so that the pressure pushes your elbows back. Hold for count of five, step back and relax. Repeat eight times.

Breathing Breathe regularly throughout the exercise.

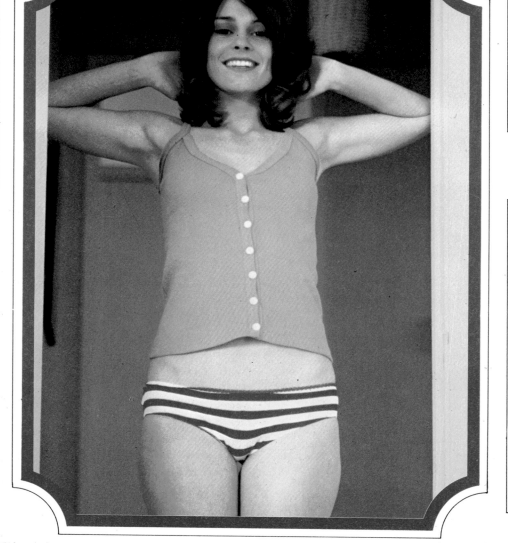

Exercise 7

Below Stand with your back to a wall; your feet about six inches from it and slightly apart. Flop forward from the hips, with head down, arms swinging freely. Now uncurl slowly, pressing your bottom against the wall and feeling each part of your spine touch the wall as you go. Your shoulders should be quite hunched as you come up, relaxing well back and down as your head touches the wall. Relax and repeat twice.

Breathing Breathe out with head hung down, in as you uncurl, and evenly as you relax in the upright position.

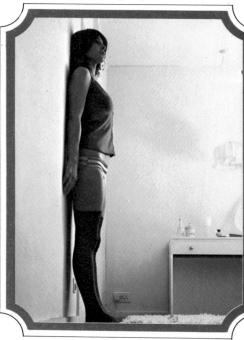

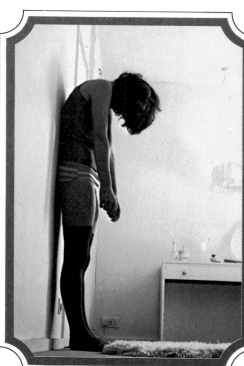

Exercise 8

Below Try to remember to do this whenever you wear a dress with a long back zipper. Step into the dress, ease your arms through the arms and stand up straight. Keeping your back straight, reach behind you with your right hand and pull the zipper up as far as you can. Reach over your left shoulder with your left hand and pull the zipper right up. You must keep your back straight throughout. Sometimes reverse the order of the hands.

Breathing Breathe regularly throughout the exercise.

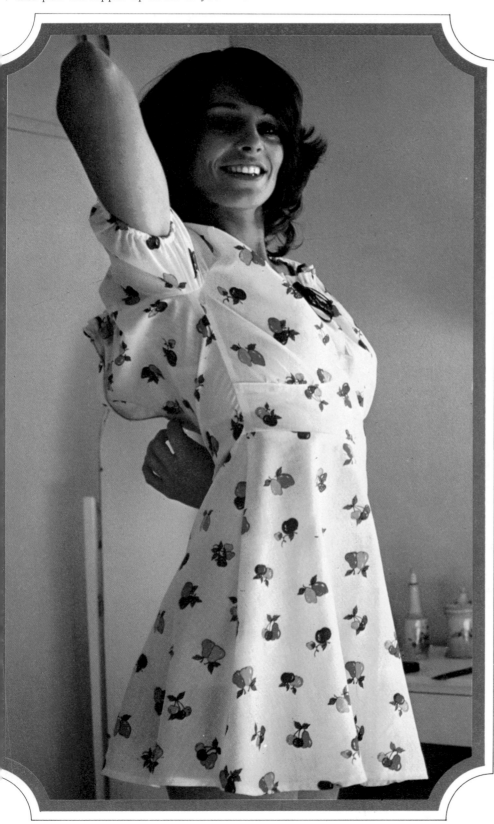

Points to note

Once you have mastered these simple posture exercises apply them to the way you carry yourself in everyday life. How you hold yourself whether in the privacy of your own home or in the office will determine the kind of impression you make on other people. Here are the points to aim for whether you are sitting, standing, walking or simply lying down.

Sitting

Your bottom should be pressed back against the back of the chair, your thigh pressed evenly on the seat and the hip-joint forming a right-angle. Your feet should be flat on the floor with the knees and ankle joints also forming right-angles. Don't cross your ankles. You should check that any chair which you sit on for long periods, especially at work, is the correct height so that knee and hip joints can form the right angle. If you're sitting in a chair at home, keep to these principles and try to avoid slumping in an armchair for long periods. Don't cross your legs—this action inevitably causes the spine to curve forwards. If you're fond of sitting on the floor, then sit cross-legged with your back straight with your hands in your lap or resting on your knees. This is the most comfortable and healthy position to adopt.

Standing

Hold your body upwards comfortably stretched, but without being stiff, so that the backbone follows its natural curves and these aren't exaggerated in any way. Balance your weight easily and evenly on both feet. Hold your hips at the same level with seat pulled in and stomach muscles held firm. Now relax shoulders and set them back a little—with your arms loosely by your sides. If you're doing everything correctly, then an imaginary vertical straight line should pass just behind your ear, through shoulders, arms, hands and legs to your ankles. This basic posture is the pose to use when you're standing still: if you have heavy parcels to hold, make sure the weight is evenly balanced. Don't cross your ankles or lean heavily on one foot. If you're waiting at a bus-stop or for a train and wish to read, then hold the book or newspaper well up so that you don't have to poke your head forward—and thus hunch your shoulders.

Walking

Adopt the standing posture. When you walk, tilt the body slightly forward as you take each step. Point your toes forward as you walk, and lift the heel of the back foot well off the ground as you transfer your weight to the front foot. Don't drag your feet or shuffle. Avoid shoes with very high heels which push all your weight onto your toes. Platform soles with ankle support can help to minimize this effect while still being fashionable. Doctors tend to prefer them to high heels. Check your reflection in shop windows occasionally to make sure you're walking correctly. Swing your arms freely, but not in an exaggerated way. Look at the path ahead, not at your feet.

Lying down·

Good posture matters—even when you're asleep. Keep your spine in good shape by avoiding high pillows, beds that are too soft or a curled up position as you sleep. After all, we spend one third of our lives in bed—so it makes sense to adopt a healthy sleeping position. If you habitually sleep with knees tucked up to chest, then your breathing is bound to be affected. In winter, warm the bed thoroughly so you won't be tempted to hunch up legs back and shoulders. The best position is flat on your back, or on your side with legs stretched straight down, arms resting lightly on the bed in front of your body. It's better to sleep without a pillow if you can—since they do help to promote double chins as well as bad posture.

Posture in Pregnancy

Don't lean back. Take the extra weight of your pregnancy on the back and legs, and support it with your thighs when you're sitting. Keep your back absolutely straight—it's far less tiring. After your baby is born, don't make the common mistake of slouching forward. Keep your shoulders back and down. When picking up your toddlers, try to remember to bend from the knees, and don't stoop. Take their weight on your legs, not on your shoulders.

The Mirror Test

Check your posture in a long mirror every morning. Stand straight, your shoulders back (but comfortable, not exaggerated), stomach and bottom tucked in. Now *look* in that mirror. Would a straight line taken from behind your ear pass vertically through shoulders, arms, legs and ankle? If you are standing correctly it should.

BENEFITS OF GOOD POSTURE

A supple spine helps to avoid backache, muscular strain and fatigue.
Shoulders back enables the lungs to breathe freely and increases resistance to disease.
Backbone upright aids digestion and frees you of heartburn, indigestion and constipation.
Feet properly used maintains circulation and avoids cramps.

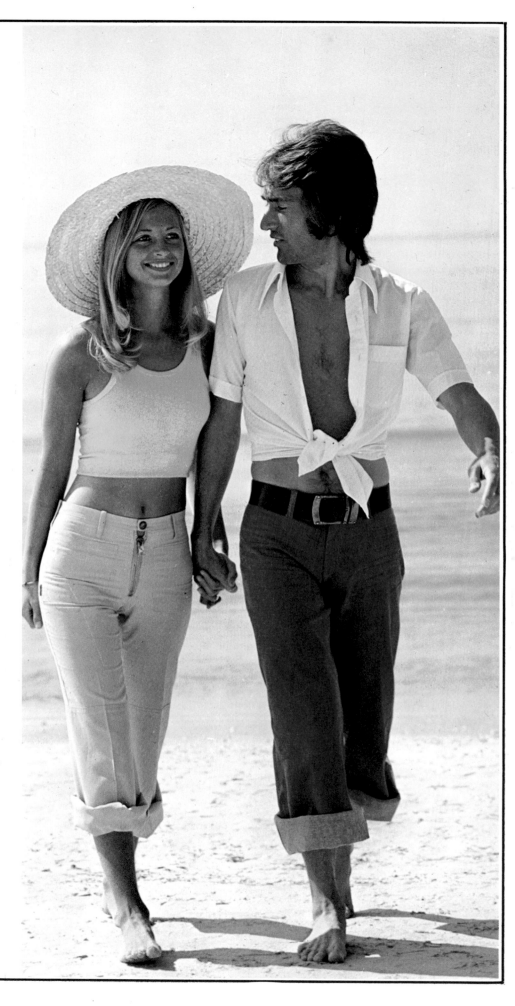

Check your breathing

Do you find exertion that is even slightly out of the ordinary leaves you short of breath? If you are out of condition, the efficiency of your lungs will be seriously impaired. Coupled with poor posture and over-weight, this could put your health seriously at risk and shorten your life.

BAD posture – shoulders forward, head drooping – obviously restricts the capacity of the lungs to take in enough life-giving air. An average adult should have a chest expansion of at least two inches and your minimum chest circumference should be at least two inches larger than your waist measurement. If you can't manage these figures, you may be in trouble. These statistics are vital – they are key figures

sequent strain all round.

Emotional reactions increase the burden, because when you're tense or excited or in some way worked up, the demand for oxygen increases and your breathing is affected. Your breath comes in short pants. What you have to realize is that shortness of breath is an ageing factor, so the sooner you start to correct any tendencies you may have in this

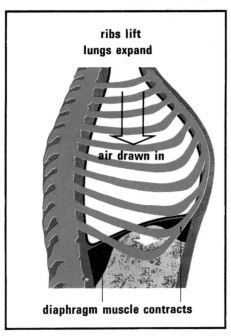

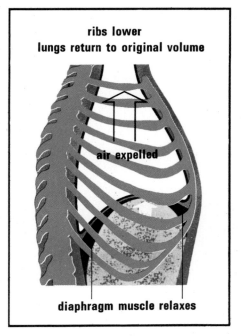

Above *When you breathe in, the ribs lift up and air is pulled into the lungs by the diaphragm muscle. If your posture is* *incorrect, however, less air will enter the lungs and you have to breathe faster— straining the whole body uselessly.*

which you must do all in your power to maintain.

For an average healthy individual, a waist measurement larger than two inches smaller than chest measurement is a danger signal, for this gives an indication of poor posture, the probability that you are overweight and that your breathing capacity is less than it should be.

Ideally, when breathing, all air in the lungs should be exchanged, but in fact this doesn't happen. What we call 'dead space' air is not completely mechanically exchanged. When you're young with a lung structure that is very elastic the joints of the ribs are still supple and the diaphragm well pressed down, 'dead space' is of little consequence. But as you grow older you suffer a general loss of elasticity and the maximum exchange of air is reduced. Bad posture enhances lack of movement and encourages shallow breathing and chest expansion is reduced. In order to compensate for this – to pump more vital oxygen into your lungs – your rate of respiration increases with con-

direction, the better chances you will have of a healthy middle and later life. With bad posture and consequent bad breathing, smoking, and a tendency to bronchitis, the dice are heavily loaded against you.

If, after only slight effort, you find yourself short of breath, you will be receiving a message from your early warning system that all is not well and that cardio-vascular troubles are on the way. Stop smoking, take regular exercise, lose excess weight and become an upright, correctly poised human being – for, taken in time, much can be done to reverse the damage. Give your lungs a chance to expand and to repair the damage they have suffered.

Polluted air can be the cause of some of these troubles, but we seem to be awakening to some of the dangers of smoke-fouled cities and legislation to prevent air pollution is now a top health priority. Long may our newly awakened concern for the quality of all aspects of our environment continue.

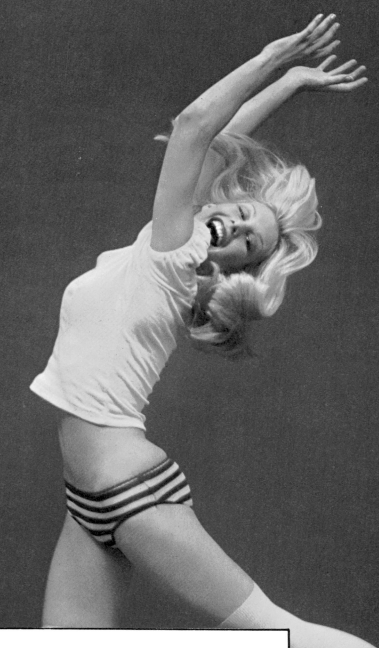

Exercise for everyone

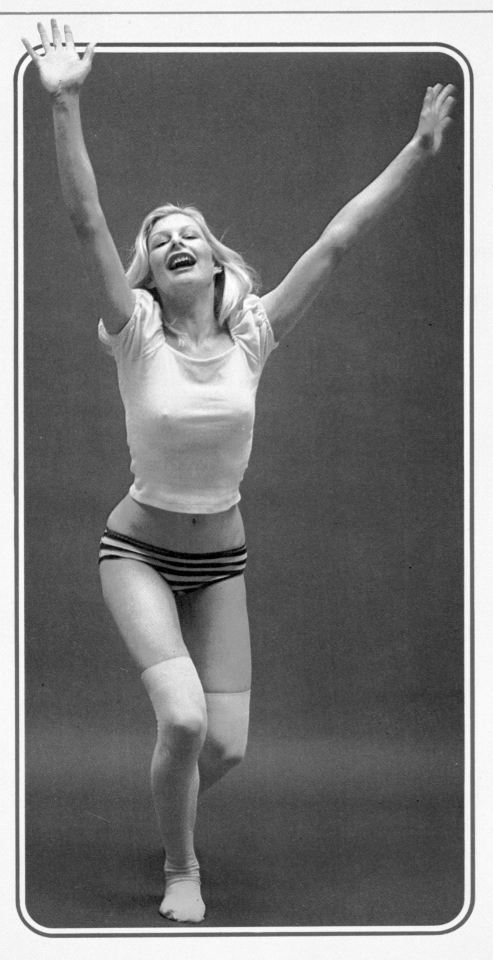

Stream- lining those problem areas—1

Dissatisfied with your shape? Who isn't? Most of us have at least one disaster zone which never seems to look good however much we diet. Too-big hips, a bulgy tummy, fatty upper-arms —they're persistent trouble spots which need tough action. Add the other 'big three'—waistline, thighs and a droopy bustline—and you have six of the worst and most common figure-faults around.

Why? Firstly, because these are six vulnerable areas where muscle tone is often weak since normal everyday activity just isn't geared to giving it work to do. In fact, our lifestyle can actually help to pile on the inches. For instance, if big hips and a sagging tummy are your main figure problems, then sitting down all day at an office desk is very likely to worsen them.

Secondly, it's an infuriating fact that pockets of fat tend to form around slack muscle. So by sitting at that office desk tucking into a cream cake you're actually adding inches in two ways!

Thirdly, figure characteristics can be hereditary. If you come from a long line of broad-hipped individuals, then there's a good chance that you're pear-shaped too. But that doesn't mean that surplus flesh and bad muscle tone can't be licked into shape. Don't use the family weakness as a 'scapegoat'.

Living with a figure problem usually means that we learn to disguise it—with clothes. A long sweater can hide a multitude of bulges; long-sleeved dresses can cover flabby upper arms; a good supporting bra can lift a drooping bustline. But, come the summer when those cosy wrappings are lifted *off*, and the problem just has to be tackled properly. It's not much fun going off on holiday with a suitcase full of long-sleeved sweaters and knee-length skirts because you look ghastly in T-shirts and tight jeans.

What's needed is an intensive campaign of action. Here's our three-point plan:

1. Recognize those faults
No need to dwell on this if you've been conscious of a sagging seat ever since you accidentally caught sight of your reflection in a shop window at the age of 10. But if you're still an innocent, then just check out your shape in front of a full-length mirror. These are the things to look for:

a) tummy-bulge—even when you're breathing *in!*

b) 'Jodhpur' handles on outsides of thighs, slack flesh on insides.

c) podgy upper arms—more than an inch of 'slack' when you grab the flesh between finger and thumb.

d) hip measurement more than three inches bigger than bust measurement—make slight allowance for 'large bone structure'.

e) a 'wandering' waistline—difficult to pinpoint exactly where it is!

THE BIG SIX

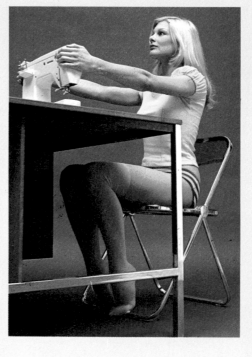

These are the most common figure-faults of all: half a dozen vulnerable body areas which *you* can trim into shape. Identify which your problem areas are— you probably know already if you're honest with yourself—then consult the chart to find the right tactics.

Bust

Main causes:
The bustline is supported by a group of muscles in the upper chest called the pectorals. *The breasts themselves contain no muscle.*

Unfortunately, the pectorals don't get much exercise—so it's necessary to make a conscious effort to keep the bustline in good shape. Many women find that they lose weight quickly from the bustline when they slim, leaving unattractive loose flesh behind. Wearing a bra is vital for any woman with a bust measurement of more than 34 inches (medium cup); otherwise those pectorals just can't cope, and sagging is inevitable.

What you can do about it:
Help the pectorals to do their job by walking and sitting with your back straight. Wear a bra—and make sure it really *does* support the breasts and has wide, comfortable shoulder straps if you have a large bust. Don't hump heavy shopping bags with the weight forward: stand up straight and take the weight on your back and legs.
Good sports: swimming, gymnastics.

Stomach

Main causes:
Like the waistline, the stomach area is particularly susceptible to sagging muscles through too much sitting and too little *natural* control. Most people just don't bother to hold stomach muscle in—and how it shows! Eating large meals stretches stomach muscles. And starting a pregnancy with weak abdominal muscles is a sure way to end up with a sagging tummy when it's all over.

What you can do about it:
Consciously hold stomach muscles in all the time—it will soon become habit. Eat smaller meals more often, instead of distending your stomach and stretching abdominal muscles unnaturally after huge 'blow-outs' once a day. *Don't* wear constricting corsetry: make those muscles work!
Good sports: gymnastics, cricket, rugby, baseball (the last three involve throwing, good exercise for tummy muscles). Dancing is also good.

Waistline

Main causes:
Constant sitting (at work, watching television) with bad posture makes the abdominal group of muscles slacken generally, adding inches to that waistline. Wearing tight belts on skirts and trousers can prevent muscles from working naturally; this is especially important for children and teenagers, who should be developing firm muscles.

What you can do about it:
Walk 'tall', holding midriff firmly in place, keeping spine erect. Sit on an upright chair, with back straight—at work and at home. Avoid very tight belts—that spare flesh has to go somewhere. Follow a good low-calorie diet and avoid excess alcohol. This is particularly important for men, who often rediscover a 'lost' waistline if they give up drinking vast quantities of beer. Whittle down the inches with a combination of diet and exercise.
Good sports: tennis, squash, golf, swimming, basketball, netball.

f) droopy bustline—whatever the measurement.

2. Determine to do something about them

Consult the chart for your plan of action and tackle the appropriate exercises. A concentrated assault on the areas concerned will give good results in quite a short time. However, you may have to change a few bad habits *permanently* and keep up specific exercises in order to make those results last. Figure-faults tend to keep returning—especially if you're in a job which involves sitting down, stooping, or other occupational hazards.

3. Stay mirror-conscious

This is one aspect of slimming which won't be helped by constant weight-checking. The scales may show a steady weight, but muscles may be slackening through lack of proper exercise. This is particularly vital after a holiday—natural activity like swimming and walking will certainly tone muscles and they'll sag quickly once that activity ceases, even though body weight may actually go *down* once you stop eating those rich holiday foods. The best check is the daily 'mirror test'. A firm, lithe figure is good to look at. Is yours?

This well designed two part Streamline Exercise Plan gives you two exercises for each problem area.
The set in part one—the model is wearing yellow—are isometric, exercises where you just contract the muscles. You can do them at home or in the office. The other set—the model is wearing blue—in the second part of the course are more energetic and demanding —but lots of fun.
All you do is determine your problem areas—there's a good chance that there are more than one and that you've a good idea what they are—and then follow the exercises given for them, one for indoors and one for outside. Do the relevant exercises from the first set for a week to get you toned up for the second part.

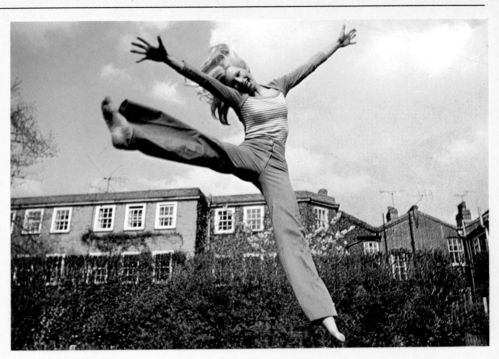

Hips and Buttocks

Main causes:
Lack of natural contraction in the buttock group of muscles, often because when we sit we rarely have anything to contract against. Squashy cushions and soft upholstery are to blame here. A bad walking action, with hips sticking out behind or to one side, can also prevent the proper 'tucking in' of the seat which helps to contract those muscles. Assembly-line workers, secretaries and office staff are the most vulnerable. Anyone who is overweight and has to support their body on over-worked buttock muscles for long periods of time will also spread in this area.

What you can do about it:
Sit on hard chairs (more comfortable for long periods, actually), throw away soft cushions and take lunch-time walks. Keep your bottom tucked in as you walk. Avoid too much driving, give up the bus and take to your feet. Walking is one of the best exercises for this area. *Good sports:* running, football, hockey, swimming.

Thighs

Main causes:
The two sets of muscles which affect the thighs most are the adductors and the abductors. The *adductors* are on the insides of the thighs, and pull the upper legs inwards. Because they're so unused, fat often accumulates around them. The *abductors* are just as neglected. Their function is to carry the leg outwards and rotate it inwards. How often do you rotate your legs inwards? Not often. No wonder thighs are a top problem area.

What you can do about it:
Walk more and run, if you can manage it. Keep thighs *taut* when you're sitting —don't let them spread all over the chair. Contract those two sets of muscles from time to time. Strangely enough this is one of the few problems that pregnancy can actually help. The extra load gives thigh muscles extra work to do, and new mums are often amazed at the firmness of their thigh muscles afterwards.
Good sports: golf, running, athletics, swimming, football.

Upper Arms and Shoulders

Main causes:
Bad posture, both sitting and standing, helps to produce 'dowagers hump', or 'typist's hunch'. Very few children are taught to sit or stand properly—and bad habits can produce a permanent stoop. Later, work can aggravate it: a salesgirl working across a low counter all day, a supermarket check-out girl who has to lean forward to take goods from a low trolley, a clerk hunched over his desk. Add to this the lack of use which the three sets of muscles in the upper arms are apt to get, and you have a problem.

What you can do about it:
Improve work conditions. Make sure you don't have to hunch—get a higher desk or a lower chair. Watch your posture and stance continuously. Take up gardening: one of the best exercises for the brachialis muscles at the front of the upper arms is shovelling earth! *Good sports:* weight-lifting, shot-put, javelin, fencing, boxing, cricket.

Streamline Exercise Plan/1

Now that you know exactly what your problem is—and what caused it—you can start to do something about it. We've devised two sets of six exercises.

The first set, based on isometrics, are simple to do and you can practice them anywhere—even in the office. For these exercises, our model wears the minimum of casual clothes—the bright yellow lifts her spirits. But you can do them in any clothes. Pick the exercises that correspond to your problem area or areas and practise them as often as possible.

If you like, you can do these by themselves for a week and then add the more energetic exercises to your routine.

The second set, the more energetic exercises, need more space. They're fun to do and are suitable for the garden, the beach or a spacious bedroom. They're in *Streamline those problem areas—2*.

Allow yourself 10 minutes every day for *each* exercise: fit it in before or after work or in your lunch-break.

With two methods of attack running simultaneously, you'll find that those problem areas will soon become toned up and the inches will start to disappear. In a week there will be a noticeable difference, but keep it up.

Exercises for home or office

Repeat these as often as possible during the day. Breathe normally and regularly throughout.

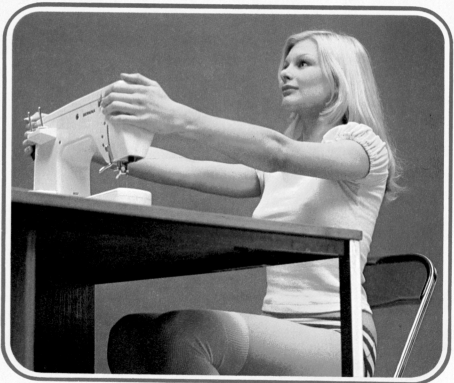

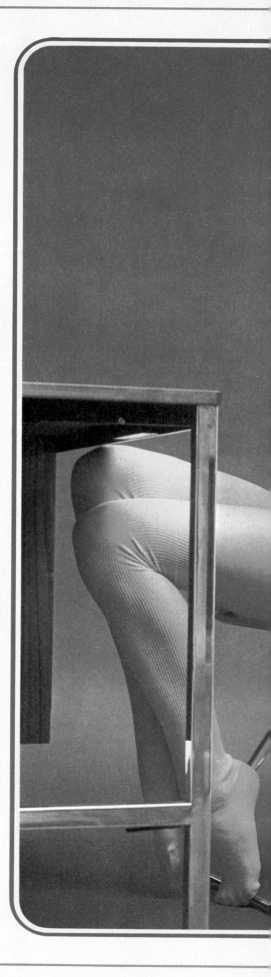

Bust

Above Sit on a straight-backed chair fairly close to a table or desk. Extend arms in front of you and place palms of hands flat each side of any solid object (sewing machine, typewriter). Keeping arms straight, push in *hard*. Hold contraction for count of six and then relax.

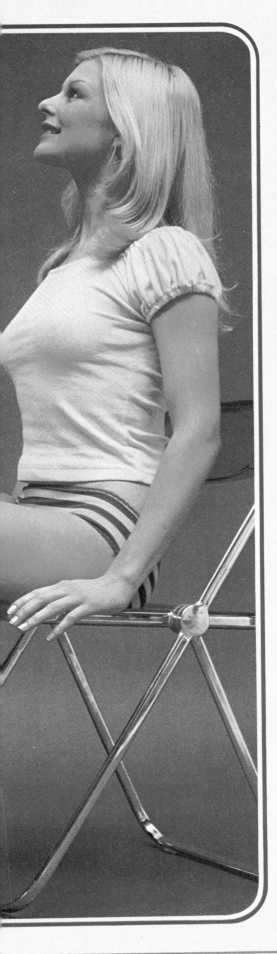

Stomach

Left Sit on the edge of a chair with knees under a table or desk. Point toes and rest them lightly on the floor. Now raise right knee to touch the underside of the table. Push upwards hard and pull stomach in at the same time, breathing *out* as you do so. Hold for count of three. Then change legs and repeat.

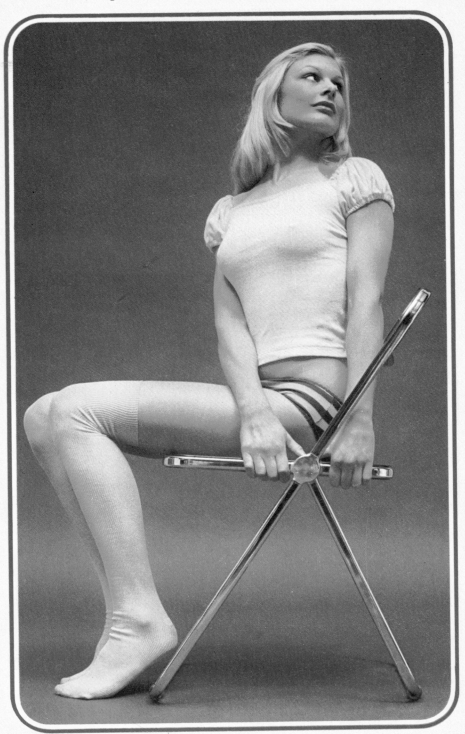

Waistline

Above Sit on a straight-backed chair, with your back straight but *away* from chair-back. Keeping legs and knees straight, grasp left side of chair-back with both hands and twist body hard to the left. Now look over left shoulder. Hold for slow count of 10 (or longer). Repeat to the right. Your buttocks must be firmly on chair all the time.

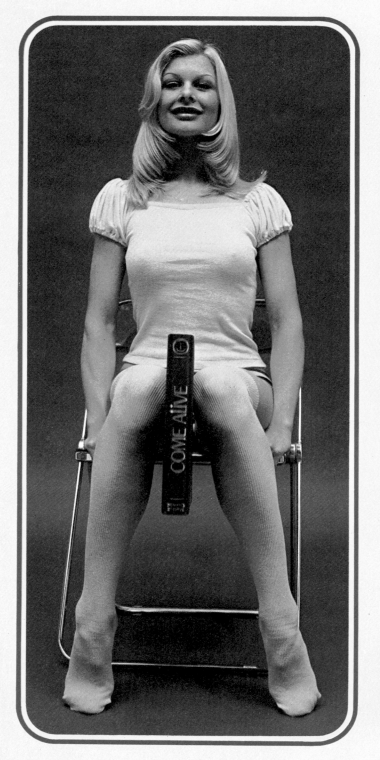

Thighs

Left Sit on a chair, holding back erect, knees straight. Now place book or magazine between your knees and squeeze together. Hold for count of six and relax. This tones *inside* thigh muscles.

Right Now sit with legs straight out in front, both feet inside a string waste-paper basket. Push out hard for count of six and relax. This tones outside thigh muscles.

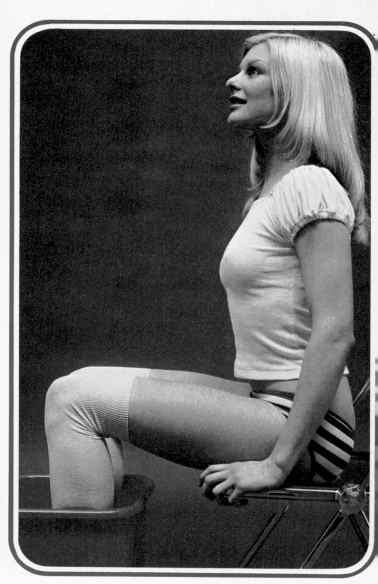

Upper Arms and Shoulders

Upper Arms and Shoulders Not shown Clench fist, bend elbow and place outside of clenched fist flat against chair-back, chair arms, wall or other resisting surface. Push hard. Hold for count of 10. Repeat.

Hips and Buttocks

Right Sit on a straight-backed chair with buttocks well back. Hold onto the seat of the chair with both hands and keep back straight. Now lift hip-bone up on left side, towards your ribcage, raising left buttock off the chair-seat as you do so. Hold for count of four. Lower and raise right side. If you're doing it properly you'll feel the 'pull' around the side of your left buttock and your right one will automatically contract to take the extra weight.

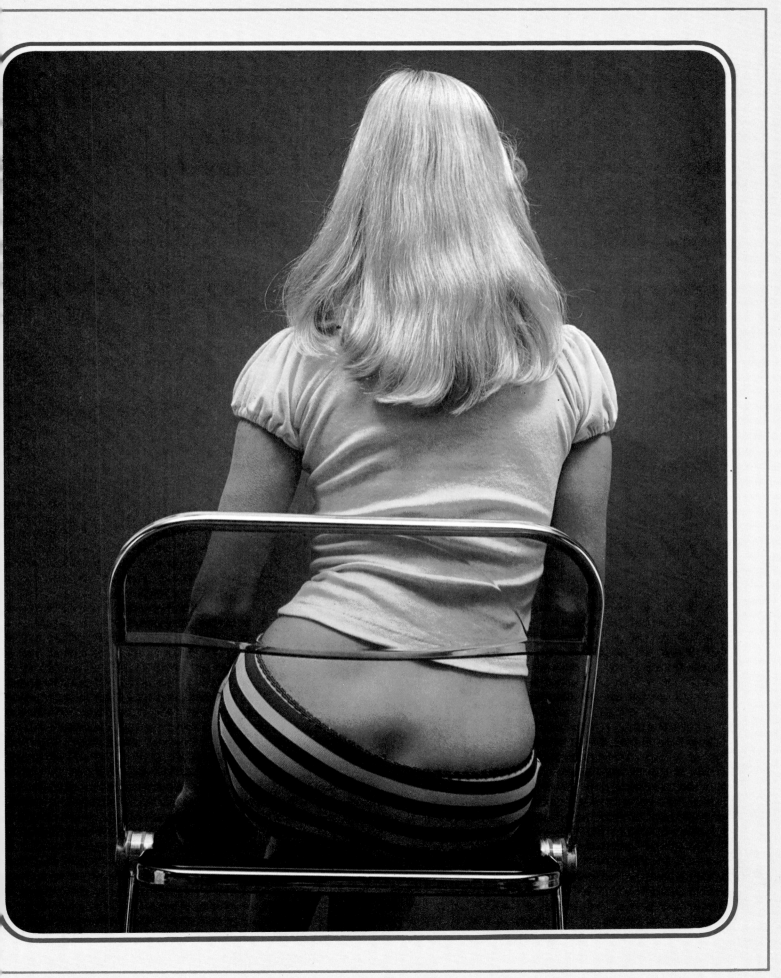

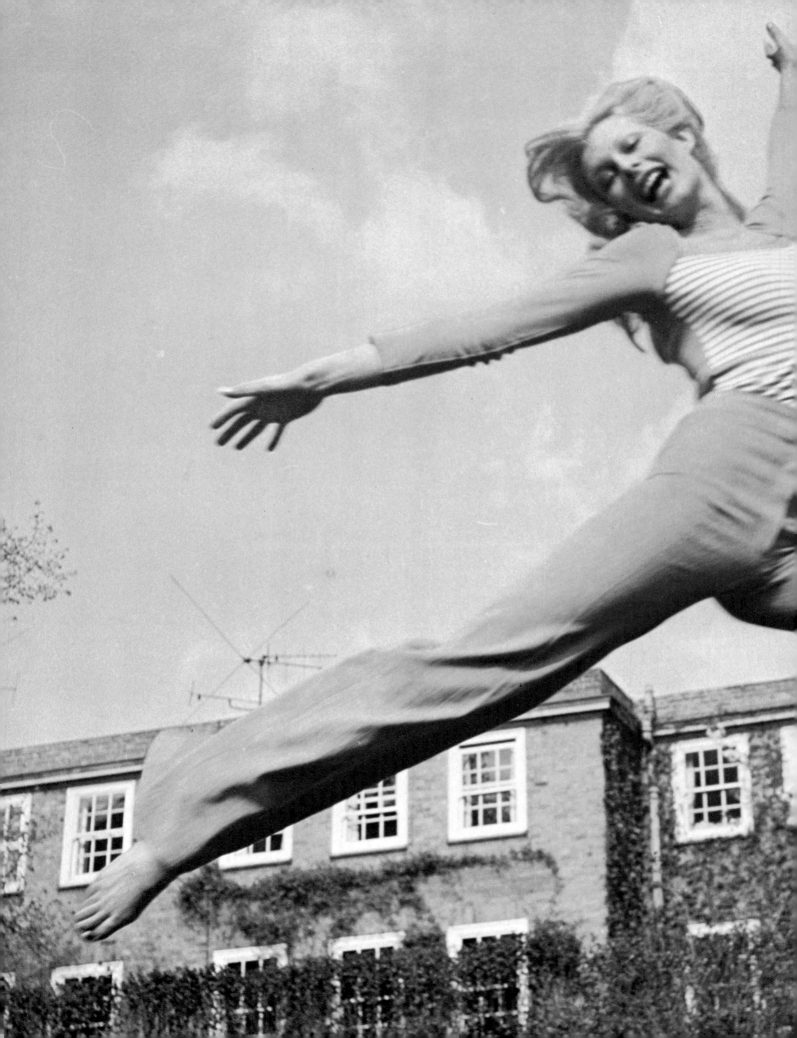

Stream— lining those problem areas-2

Lose as you choose with the second set of Streamline Spot-Reduction exercises. Fit them in before or after work, or during your lunch hour. Or, if you're at home, just take a break in the day's routine—and watch the inches glide away.

First be honest with yourself—you're the only one who can decide which areas need streamlining. Then take a look at the exercises designed for those areas and start practising.

You'll need space to allow you to move around—a garden, the beach or a large

Streamline your way to a firm, lithe figure with as little as ten minutes exercise a day. You lose as you choose with the spot-reduction plan.

bedroom is fine. And wear loose-fitting clothing. The exercises are straight-forward and take little effort—but you do want to be able to move freely.

Ten minutes a day for each exercise are all it takes—the results will soon start to show. And for maximum effect you should combine them with isometric exercises from the first set. These are so simple and unobtrusive you can do them anywhere—even while you're working.

And remember, those inches are waiting to creep back again so, once you've started, keep up the plan.

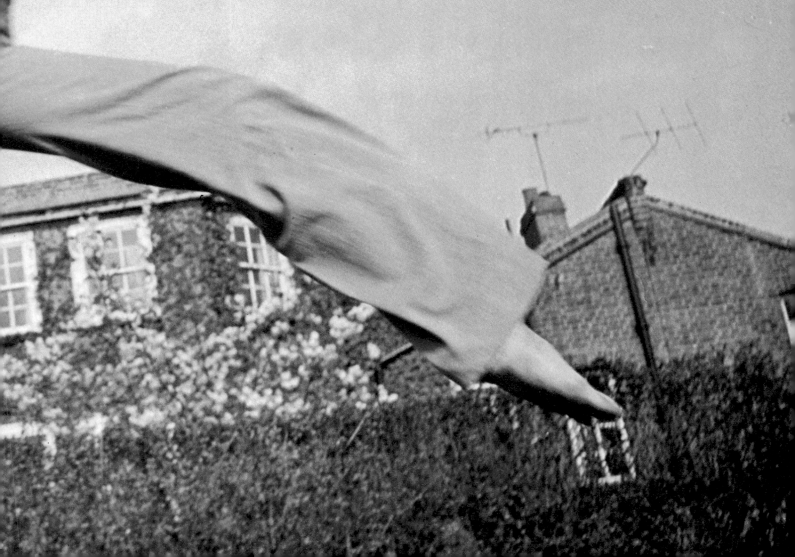

Streamline Exercise Plan/2

Pick out the exercises for your problem areas and practise them every day. Combine these movements with the static isometric exercises from the first set and you will virtually be able to watch the inches melt away. Both sets of exercises have been designed by SALLY DENHAM, F.S.B.Th., to give you maximum benefit with minimum strain.

Exercise for out of doors

Practise each of 'your' streamlining exercises for just 10 minutes a day. Follow the instructions about breathing in time with the movements.

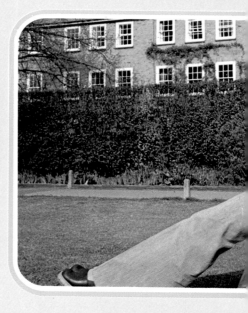

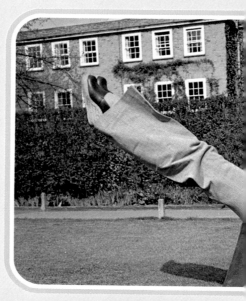

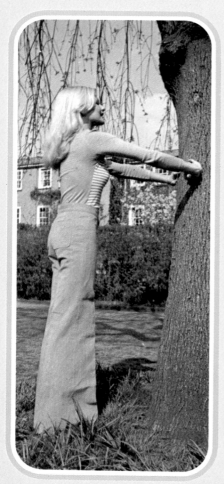

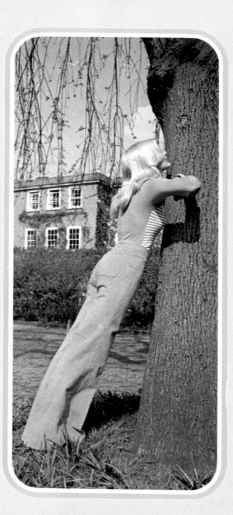

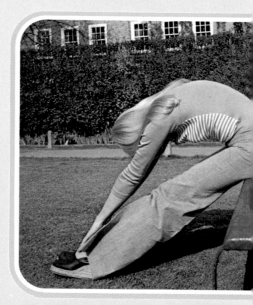

Bust

Above Stand straight, arms-distance away from a wall or tree. Place palms of hands against the wall, hands turned inwards with fingers a little way apart. Arms should be at shoulder level. Now, lean right forward, bending elbows and keeping back straight. Hold just *before* your nose touches the wall.

Remain in this position for a count of eight, then straighten up slowly. Repeat several times.

Breathing Breathe out at starting position, in as you lean forward, regularly at the held position and out again as you straighten up.

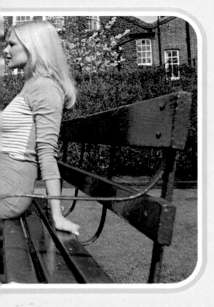

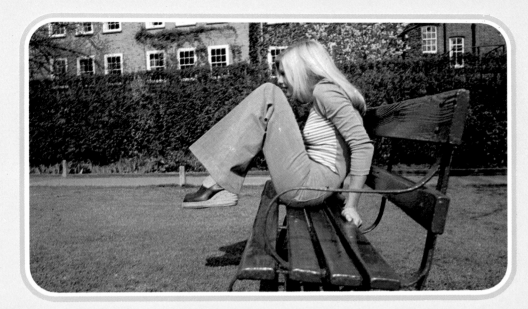

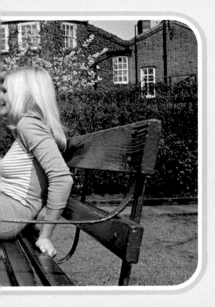

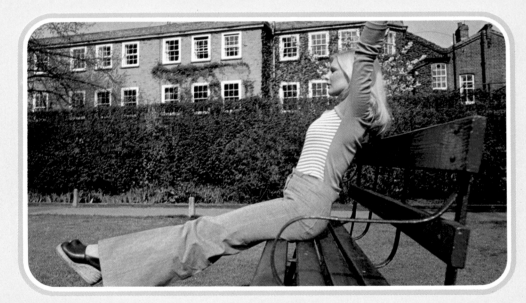

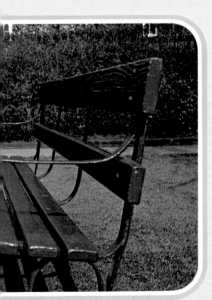

Stomach

Above Sit on the edge of a garden bench or chair, supporting your weight on your hands behind you. Now stretch out legs, point toes and raise feet just above the ground. **2** Slowly bend knees to touch chin (or almost): **3** Then stretch legs upwards at an angle of 45° to the body, keeping your back straight. **4** Gently lower legs, bringing arms forward and keeping head tucked between them as you do so. **5** Touch toes with both hands. Repeat.

Breathing Breathe in at start of movement, out as you bring knees to touch chin, in just before you stretch legs, then out and in again just before you bend down to touch toes. Exhale as you go down.

Streamlining your figure means watching your diet as well as taking exercise. You can't hope to melt away inches while piling in calories. Take a sensible approach to eating, that's all you need to do. If you're slimming already carry on with your diet—the exercises will help your figure problem at the same time as you lose weight.
If you are slightly overweight think about trying a special low calorie diet to back up the exercises. In any case, check what you're eating —a healthy diet is vital to a lively look.

Waist

Below Stand behind a garden bench or chair with right hand resting on the bench-back, feet slightly apart. Now bend forward and ease feet back slightly so that back is kept quite straight. Swing left arm down to touch right foot. Then swing arm upwards and backwards, following arm's direction with your head. Repeat 15 times, then repeat movement with your right arm.

Breathing Breathe in at start of exercise, breathe out as you swing down, in again as you swing up.

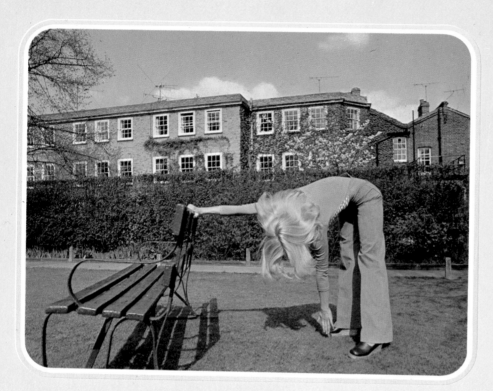

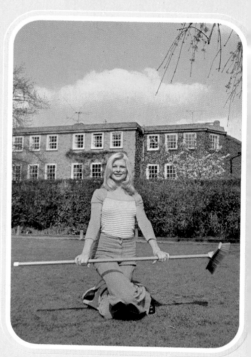

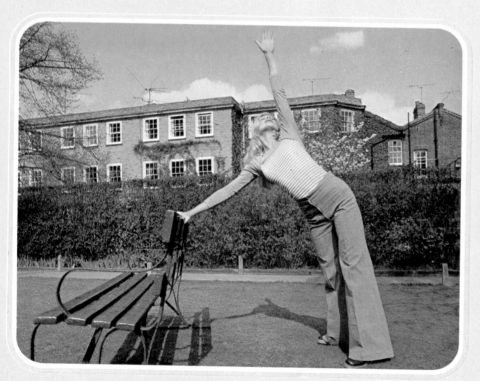

Thighs

Above Stand straight, feet together, with a broom handle or mop on the ground in front of you. Move left leg well behind right leg and bob down in a 'curtsying' action to sit on right buttock. Pick up broom with both hands apart. Now stand up using broom to help balance—but without using your hands. Raise broom above your head, squat down on haunches, and replace broom in starting position. Repeat with right leg just behind left leg. Repeat several times.

Breathing Breathe in, before you start, out as you bob down, in again as you stretch up, out as you squat.

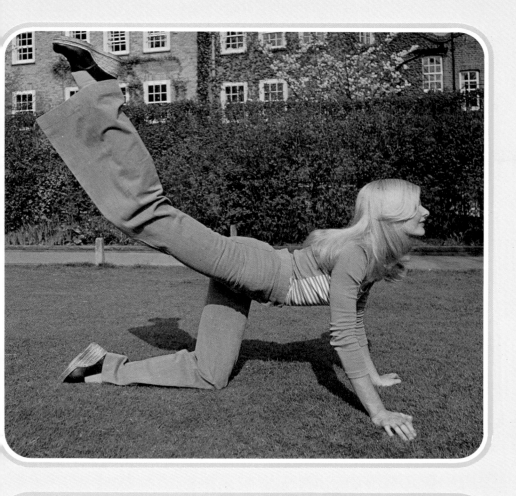

Hips and Buttocks

Left Kneel on grass or floor on all fours with back straight.
A. Lift right leg straight up behind you and make big circles *inwards*, rotating from the thigh. Repeat five times.
B. Now swing leg out at the side, keeping it up at hip level. Rapidly bend and stretch knee twice. Lower to starting position and repeat whole movement with left leg.

Breathing Take a deep breath before exercise, then breathe regularly throughout.

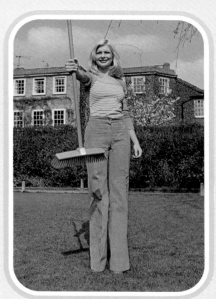

Upper Arms and Shoulders

Above Stand straight with broom or mop on the grass in front of you. Bend knees, keeping back straight and grasp broom with right hand about half way up the handle. Straighten up and raise arm to shoulder level. Punch elbow back, keeping broom vertical as you do so. Bring broom forward. Then pass or throw to left hand and repeat. Repeat several times.

Breathing Breathe in before bending knees, then breathe out. In again as you straighten, then regularly throughout rest of exercise.

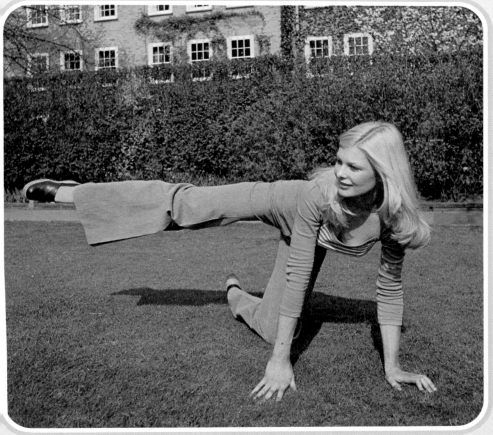

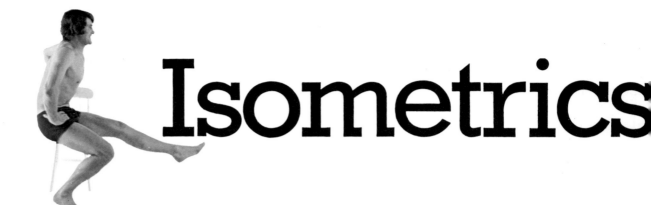

Isometrics

"One minute a day is all you need spend to develop your strength." Isometrics has great appeal for those people who know the value of physical fitness but don't want to spend the time or money which is frequently necessary to follow a comprehensive exercise programme.

Why, in that case, has isometrics not become more popular? Is it merely because people feel they must suffer and lose something, in time, sweat or money, to become fit, or does the system of isometrics itself have inherent limitations and disadvantages? The answer is simple. The successful application of isometrics is restricted to only one specific area of fitness—that of strength and muscular development. This does not mean, however, that isometrics should be instantly rejected by those people who think they are already sufficiently strong and muscular.

There is nothing new or difficult about isometrics. We are all actually performing isometrics every day of our lives. A muscle or group of muscles is working isometrically when you hold any fixed position. When you stand, for example, your postural muscles—in your feet, calves, thighs, hips and trunk—work in this way. The muscles in your arms and shoulders, on the other hand, will be relaxed and therefore not working isometrically, since they are neither being contracted nor working to hold a fixed position.

If, however, your arms were raised sideways to shoulder level and held there, then your shoulder muscles would be working isometrically to hold this fixed position against the pull of gravity. As an exercise programme, isometrics are merely an extension of this principle.

Muscles, of course, have functions other than isometric. The most common function is to provide locomotion, the movements of the limbs and trunk. When you sit down, for example, your thigh and hip muscles stretch and lengthen, thus allowing your legs and hip joints to flex so that you can lower your hips to rest on the chair. When you stand up the same group of leg and hip muscles must work by contracting and shortening in order to

extend your knees and hip joints and raise the weight of your body back to its upright position.

During the lowering and raising, the muscles are working isotonically. Isotonic action is dynamic. It occurs when muscles change length to produce or permit body actions such as lifting, walking, running, swimming and cycling. You cannot make a movement without isotonic action by the muscles which are involved in that movement.

When you embark on a course of isometric and isotonic exercises, you are

Anyone can do it, it can be done anywhere, and it costs nothing. So why isn't isometrics the most popular of exercise programmes?

not doing anything unusual. All day long you do a mixture of isotonic and isometric muscle contractions, whenever you move or hold a fixed position. Naturally there are countless degrees of isometric intensity. These range from merely holding the weight of your forearm while the elbow is bent, to exerting full muscular force against an immovable object, which is called *maximal isometric contraction*.

There are hundreds of degrees of variation between minimal contractions —those which merely maintain the static position of the limbs or body—and maximal contractions. If you hold a pencil in your hand, then a book, followed by a heavier book and so continue, gradually increasing the weight, the opposing resistance of your biceps and the other muscles in your arm also increases. The intensity and, therefore, the effectiveness of isometric exercises depends on the amount of pressure you apply when pulling, pushing or trying to turn an immovable object. This principle enables a person using isometrics to gradually progress from gently applied effort to maximal force.

The success of isometrics as a strength-builder is dramatically illustrated by the story of Alexander Zass, a Russian

strongman who performed in the thirties. As a prisoner of war, Zass had exercised his muscles by pulling and pushing against the bars and other immovable objects.

Zass later travelled around the world and, in both circuses and music halls, demonstrated his amazing ability by bursting chains around his chest and bending iron bars across his thighs, neck and knees.

Isometrics certainly succeeds in developing strength in those muscles which are involved in exerting force. But the application of that strength is then limited to particular functions. Assume, for example, that you have an old-fashioned sash window, the type which slides up and down, and that it is stuck. The top part of the bottom frame is at mid-chest level. Putting the heels of both hands under it you push up, a movement which would involve your shoulder and arm muscles. If you continued doing this every day for several weeks, you might finally move or loosen the window, or break the frame—or even damage your hands.

If, after weeks of exercising these muscles at that particular point in their range of movement, you tried to open another window—this time one whose top frame was much higher, perhaps at forehead level—then the strength developed by previously pressing at chest level will be diminished, despite the fact that basically the same muscles are working. This is because your limbs and joints are now at different angles and different muscle fibres are involved. To be able to apply your potential strength at both chest and forehead levels you would need to practise at both levels. Specific isometric exercises will only develop certain muscles for particular tasks.

Although isometrics are unquestionably successful in developing strength and muscles, there is little chance of achieving spectacular results in other spheres, such as in the efficiency of the heart and lungs. And, when most people discuss fitness, they are referring to the ability to exert themselves physically without becoming breathless, and to

& Isotonics

recover quickly from exertion. The development of this kind of fitness is brought about only by dynamic movement, by isotonics, usually against fairly moderate resistance, and repeated many times so that the heart and lungs have to work increasingly harder and longer as training progresses. The same applies to the improvement of joint mobility and speed —they can only be bettered by isotonics.

The man mainly responsible for provoking interest in isometrics was Professor E. A. Mueller, and later his colleague Dr. Theodor Hettinger, at the Max Planck Institute at Dortmund in West Germany. Although Mueller's work in isometric research, published in the mid-fifties, was in no way concerned with athletics or sportsmen, it fired the imagination of physical educationalists, coaches and athletes throughout the world.

Hundreds of articles, books and lectures were produced, but in sport the enthusiasm dropped fairly rapidly to a more sensible level. Isometrics was merely regarded as another training method to be used under certain circumstances, another tool in the coach's bag.

Many specialists, in various fields, were already familiar with the advantages of isometrics—and the dangers. Known to remedial gymnasts, physiotherapists and doctors as "static contractions," isometrics have been used in hospitals and rehabilitation centres since before the First World War. At that time it was found that by tightening or contracting muscles their tone was improved and muscle strength was developed or maintained. Isometrics are still widely and successfully used in physiotherapy.

The degree of success in isometrics for anyone will always depend on several factors. The planned efficiency of the exercise course and the effort and determination of the exerciser are of greatest importance. And, as with any exercise programme, adequate sleep and a proper diet will contribute to its success. But the results, in the development of strength and muscle tone, particularly in terms of the minimal time involved in exercising, certainly make isometrics worthwhile.

What of the dangers? Research has produced evidence to show that maximal (full force) isometrics can be dangerous for the person who is unfit and overweight, or for those people who suffer from high or low blood-pressure. Even the younger person who has had little real physical exercise for some time must be careful, and should obey the same elementary rules.

Always begin your isometric sessions with a few isotonic warming-up exercises. These exercises require no equipment and are done standing. Always be sure that your pulse rate is raised before starting your isometrics. Without this precaution isometrics would push your pulse rate up without warning, and this would be dangerous for people with any cardiovascular weakness.

During the first few days of doing isometric exercises be sure that the force you apply to your pulling or pushing is well below your maximum effort. You should begin by applying force for not longer than two seconds in each position, and add one second each time until you reach the stage when you are exercising

We perform isometrics and isotonics every day of our lives. By elaborating on this elementary principle you can increase your strength.

three to five days each week for contractions of six seconds with a force some 30 per cent below maximum. After several weeks of training you can apply maximum force to each position of contraction once every fourth exercise period.

If you are more than 30 years old and feel that you have been badly out of condition for some time and become easily tired, it is advisable to first consult your doctor and then begin only with light isotonic exercises until your fitness improves. After a few weeks, you can then progress to low-force isometrics.

What, then, are the general conclusions about isometrics? Researchers, including Mueller and Hettinger, are agreed that the intensity and duration of isometric muscle contraction is important in the development of strength. They also believe that the minimal amount of applied isometric force must be at least one-third of maximal isometric force if worthwhile results are to be obtained. About half of the maximal force possible produces really good results considering the time and effort involved.

It is unnecessary and undesirable to hold the contraction until the muscle or muscles are fatigued. It is advisable to give up long before this stage is reached, and six seconds should be considered maximal. One isometric contraction for the recommended time once each day is sufficient to produce the best results, and strength gained over weeks or months can be maintained for a long time by one or two exercise periods a week. Isometrics is essentially a time-saver.

The central purpose of isometric exercises is to develop strength in the various muscles activated by each of the static positions assumed in your exercise course. These exercises do not develop real endurance in terms of the efficiency of the heart and lungs, nor are they designed for improvement in joint mobility or speed. These latter qualities are best achieved by isotonic exercises. Even when endurance is your aim, however, a small selection of isometric exercises in the middle of your schedule can be beneficial.

The idea of developing strength, and therefore the idea of isometrics, may not appeal to some women. Their reaction tends to be one of "I get strong enough doing housework." Yet, if women use isometrics sensibly, they will become stronger without becoming more muscular. The housework will then seem much easier, and pleas to the man of the household to open a jar or a window would become less frequent.

The specially designed course which follows will enable both men and women to reap the benefits from a system that is simple, quick, and inexpensive. In accordance with the medically proven view that isometrics should not be done on their own, the course includes easy but effective isotonics as a corollary to the main isometric course.

Isometrics/ Isotonics-1

Free-standing Exercises

These warming-up exercises, to be done by both men and women, are designed to increase mobility in all the joints so that the muscles can then move with ease and freedom over the greatest distance. The exercises should be done rhythmically with an easy but strong and long-stretching movement, without vigorous jerks. Repeat each one 10 times on the first day and build up gradually to 20.

Arm-circling

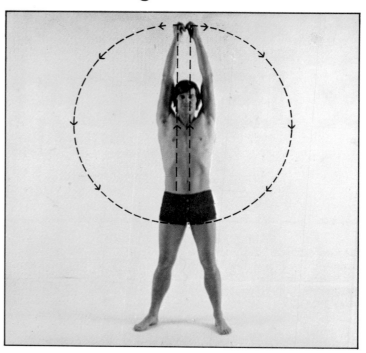

Stand with your feet wide apart and your arms at your sides. Breathing freely, raise your arms forwards and then upwards, directly above your head. Lower your arms in an arc, pulling backwards, and bring them round to the starting position.

Chin-high Kicking

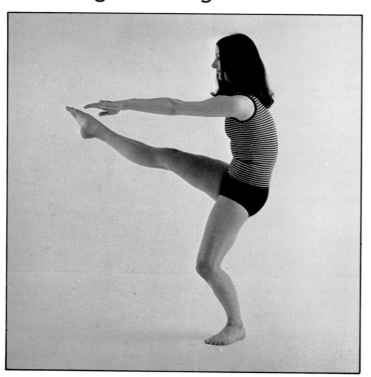

Stand with your feet together and your arms stretched out in front of you at shoulder height. Inhale. Kick forwards and upwards towards your hands, first with your right foot and then with your left. Let the standing leg bend slightly as you kick. Exhale as you lower your kicking leg.

Side-bending

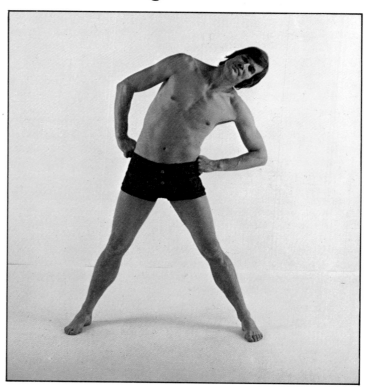

Stand with your feet wide apart and your hands on your hips, with your elbows pointing sideways. Breathing freely, bend your body to the left, making sure that your head and neck tilt with it. Then bend to the right.

Foot-reaching

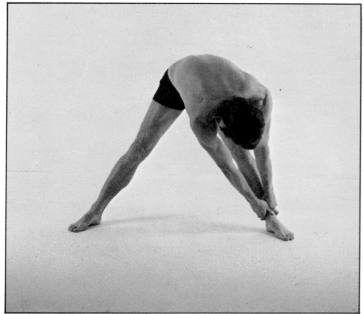

Stand with your feet wide apart and both hands on your left thigh. Inhale. Exhaling, bend forwards and sideways and slide your hands down the front of your leg. Let your spine bend without force, and let your head hang with your neck muscles relaxed. Return to an upright position, inhale, and repeat with your right leg.

Trunk-rotating

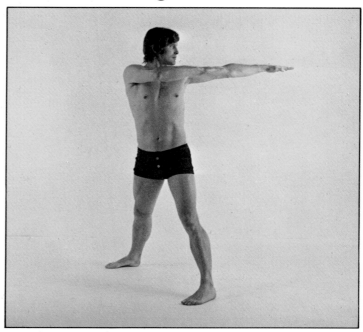

Stand with your feet wide apart and your arms raised in front of you at shoulder level. Breathing freely, turn your head, shoulders and arms to the left, keeping your hips still. Let your right arm bend at the elbow. Swing immediately to the right side and repeat.

Isometric

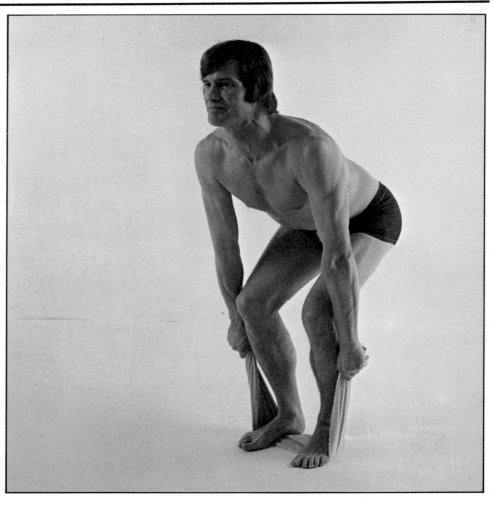

The Power Pull

Develops strength in the legs, hips, back, shoulders and arms. This exercise should only be done by men

Stand on a folded bath towel with your feet about 8 inches apart and grip the ends about 10 inches from the floor. Your knees should be bent at right-angles, your arms and back straight. Keeping your head up, pull up strongly (but not with maximal force) for two seconds. Relax. Do not repeat.

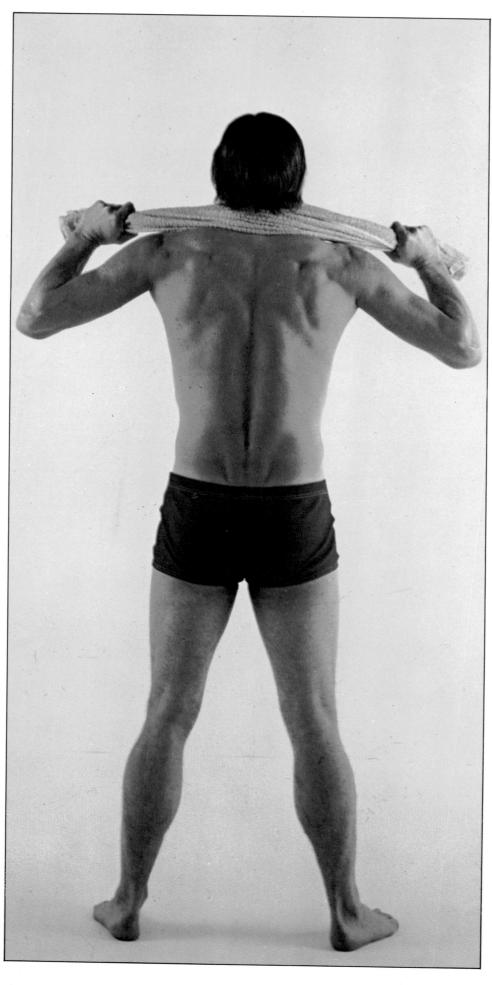

The Shoulder Press

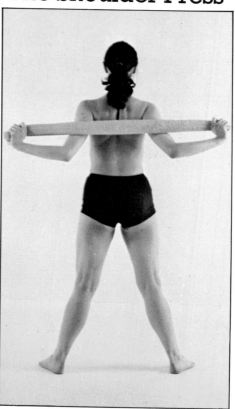

Strengthens and develops the arms and shoulders
Hold the folded towel behind your back. Pull outwards strongly with both hands for two seconds. Do not repeat.
Women will find it easier and more beneficial to hold the towel nearer the ends and pull it across a lower part of the back. Whichever you choose, make sure that each time you exercise you hold the towel in the same position.

The Cushion Crush

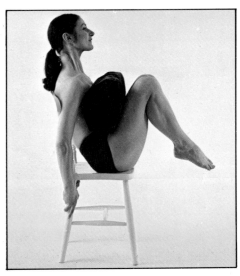

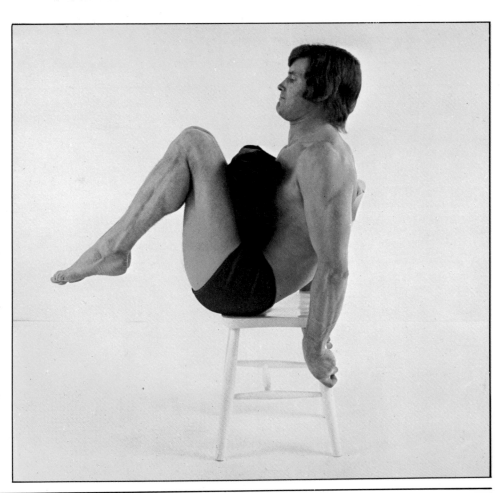

Strengthens and develops the stomach muscles and the thighs
Sit near the front edge of a sturdy straight chair and rest a cushion on the top of your thighs. Grip the sides or legs of the chair firmly with your hands and, with your knees bent, raise your thighs. Pressing strongly, try to crush the cushion between your thighs and your stomach. Hold for two seconds. Do not repeat.

Isotonic
Stationary Running

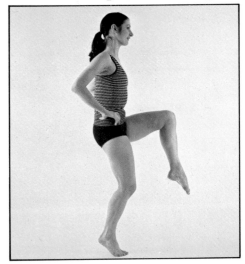

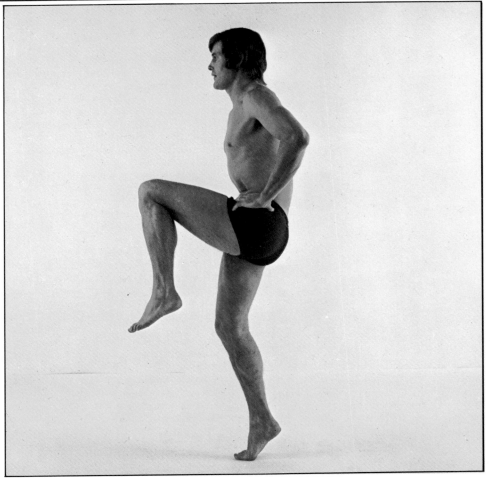

Develops efficiency of the heart and lungs and improves general fitness
Start in a standing position with your hands on your waist. Breathing freely, run on the spot on your toes. The height your knees go will depend on your fitness, but it is beneficial to go as high as possible. Begin with 30 seconds and increase by 10 seconds each day.

Isometrics/Isotonics-2

The second part of our specially designed course includes three isometric exercises —static muscular contractions where your muscles work to hold a fixed position. Only one of these exercises, The Arm Support, should be done by women.

It is important that before you begin the isometrics you mobilize all your joints by warming up with the free-standing exercises. You should follow the isometrics with an isotonic exercise—where the muscles lengthen and shorten to allow movement. The isotonic exercise for this part is the star jump.

These exercises are to be done every day for one week. It would be most beneficial if, after completing the free-standing exercises, you do the isometric exercises from the first part of the course before proceeding with the new ones. There is, however, no harm in doing only the following exercises for one week then the exercises on pages 54-56 for a week, and then combining all the exercises at the beginning of your fourth week.

Over several weeks you may gradually extend the exercises—both in the length of time the positions are held (up to six seconds) and of the force applied (up to maximal isometric force). After six weeks or so you will be able to do all the exercises included in the course, holding each one at maximal force for six seconds. Do not exceed this time however.

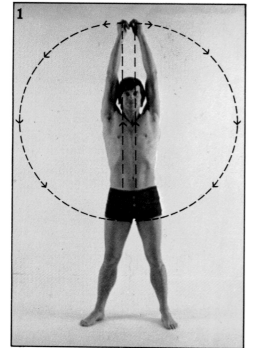

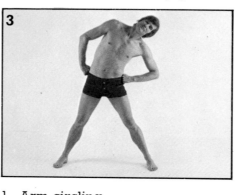

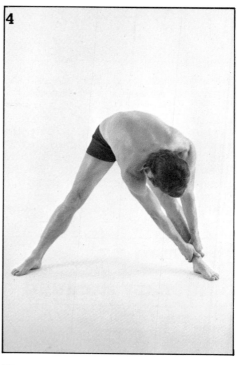

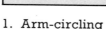

1. Arm-circling
Stand with your feet wide apart and your arms at your sides. Breathing freely, raise your arms forwards and then upwards, directly above your head. Lower your arms in an arc, pulling backwards, and bring them around to the starting position.

2. Chin-high Kicking
Stand with your feet together and your arms stretched out in front of you at shoulder height. Inhale. Kick forwards and upwards towards your hands, first with your right foot and then with your left. Let the standing leg bend slightly. Exhale as you lower your kicking leg.

3. Side-bending
Stand with your feet wide apart and your hands on your hips, with your elbows pointing sideways. Breathing freely, bend your body to the left, making sure that your head and neck tilt with it. Then bend to the right.

4. Foot-reaching
Stand with your feet wide apart and both hands on your left thigh. Inhale. Exhaling, bend forwards and sideways and slide your hands down the front of your leg. Let your spine bend without force, and let your head hang with your neck muscles relaxed. Return to an upright position. Inhale and repeat with your right leg.

5. Trunk-rotating
Stand with your feet wide apart and your arms raised in front of you at shoulder level. Breathing freely, turn your head, shoulders and arms to the left, without moving your hips. Let your right arm bend at the elbow. Swing immediately to the right side and repeat.

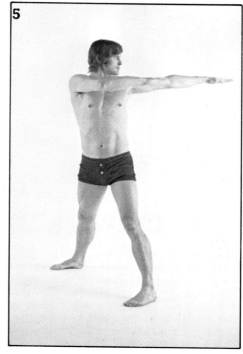

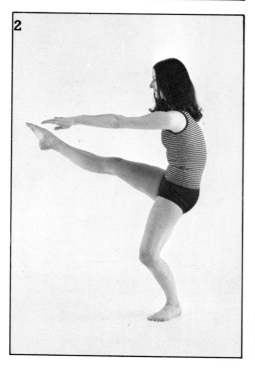

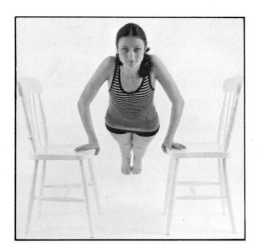

The Arm Support

Strengthens and develops the arm, shoulder and chest muscles
If you are out of condition use a fairly high table for support when you begin this exercise, and gradually substitute lower supports as your strength increases. Men will be able to use a lower support than women and should be able to hold a lower position.
Using two sturdy chairs or a low table, support your body on your toes and hands. Keeping your body straight, lower yourself as far as possible by bending your arms. Hold for two seconds. Do not repeat.

Isometric

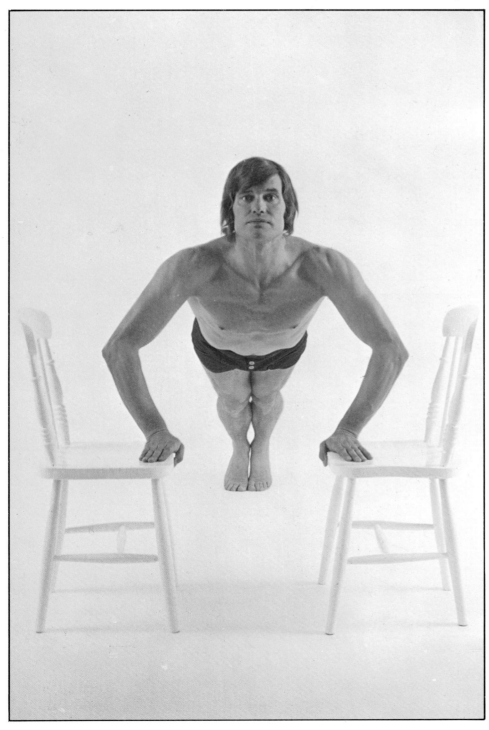

The Vertical Pull

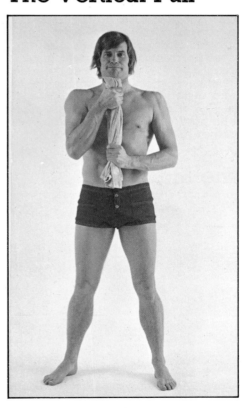

Strengthens and develops the muscles in the arms
This exercise is to be done only by men.
Stand with your feet apart. Hold a folded towel with your hands about 12 inches apart, your right hand under your chin and your left hand in front of your stomach. Pull strongly upwards with your right hand and down with your left for two seconds.
Change hands and repeat.

Isometric

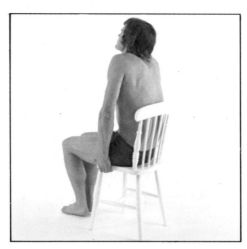

The Shoulder Pull

Develops the muscles in the shoulders and neck.
This exercise should be done only by men.
Sit well back on a sturdy chair and grip the sides of the seat with your hands. Keeping your back straight, pull upwards, raising your shoulders up towards your ears, without moving your head. Do not exert full force. Hold for two seconds. Do not repeat.

The Reach Press

Develops and strengthens the muscles in the arms, shoulders, chest and stomach.
This exercise is to be done only by men.
Lie face down on the floor with your arms outstretched in front of you and your feet slightly apart and resting on your toes. Raise your head and chest off the floor as far as possible and, with your arms straight and your head well up, press down firmly with your hands. Hold for two seconds. Do not repeat. After several weeks you may succeed in raising your trunk clear of the floor. But this should not be attempted until your strength has considerably increased.

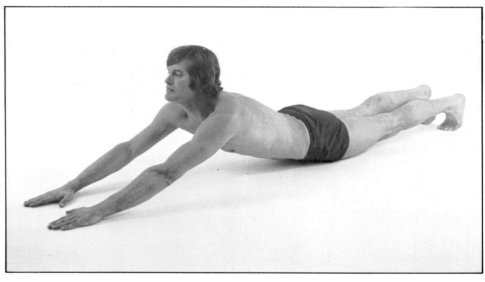

The Side Pull

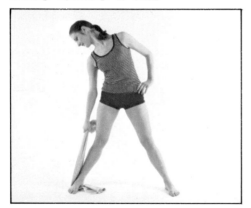

Develops and strengthens the muscles in the neck, shoulders, arms, sides and legs.
Stand with your feet well apart. Put one end of a folded towel under the heel of your right foot, and grip the other end so that your hand is just above knee level. Put your left hand on your hip. Keeping your head, shoulder, arm and foot in a vertical straight line, pull strongly on the towel, as though you were trying to stretch it, for two seconds. Relax. Repeat on your left side.

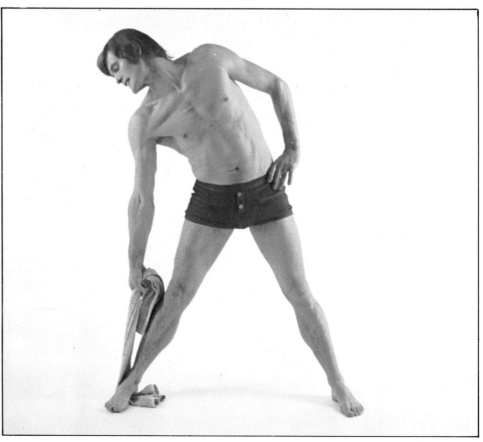

Isotonic

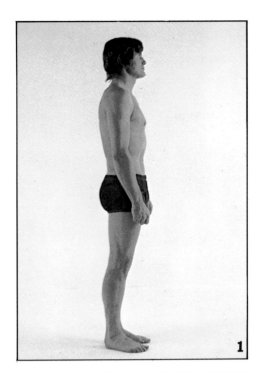

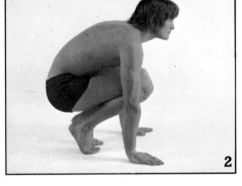

Burpees

Develops general fitness.
This exercise is to be done only by men. Women should substitute either stationary running or star jumps.
1. Stand with your arms relaxed by your sides. **2.** Bend your knees until you are crouching with your hands on the floor in front of your feet. **3.** Jump backwards with your legs until your body is in the front support position.
Return to the crouch position immediately and stand up.
At first do this exercise slowly and repeat six to 10 times. Then gradually build up until you are doing the exercise as one uninterrupted movement up to 30 times.

Stationary Running

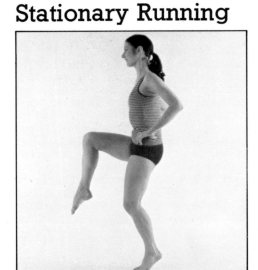

Develops efficiency of the heart and lungs and improves general fitness.
Start in a standing position with your hands on your waist. Breathing freely, run on the spot on your toes. The height your knees go will depend on your fitness, but it is beneficial to go as high as possible. Begin with 30 seconds and increase by 10 seconds each day.

Star Jumps

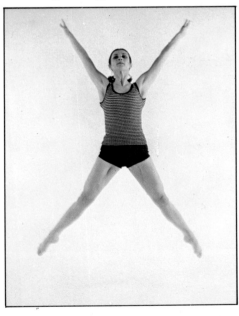

Develops the heart and lungs and improves general fitness.
Stand with your feet a few inches apart, your knees slightly bent and your arms at your sides with the palms of your hands facing inwards. Leap upwards, bringing your arms well up and outwards, and pushing your feet out sideways.
Repeat eight to 10 times and gradually increase to 30 times.

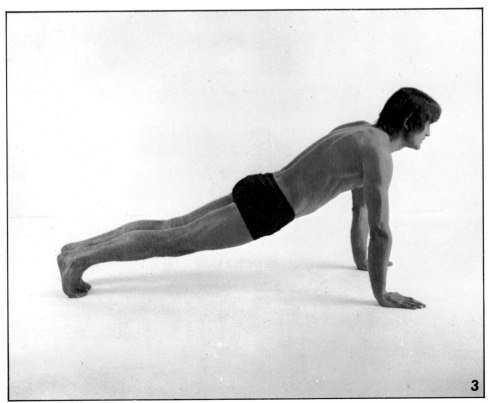

Continuation

This course has been specifically designed as an introduction to isometrics. One of the great advantages of isometrics, however, is the endless variety of exercises that can be done with little preparation (except the obligatory warming-up) and with simple equipment. After completing the introductory course you can add your own exercises.

The following exercises, using a broom handle, for pushing and pulling, are four more exciting variations you can try.

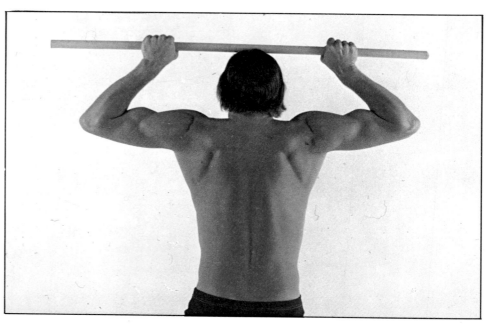

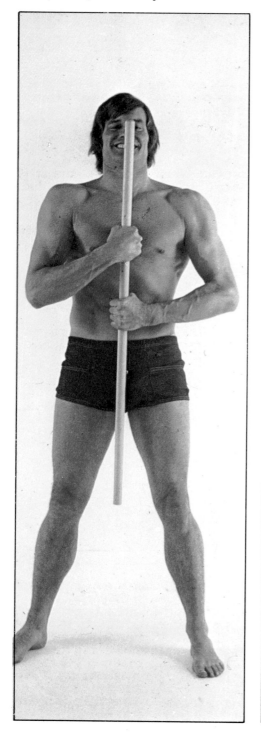

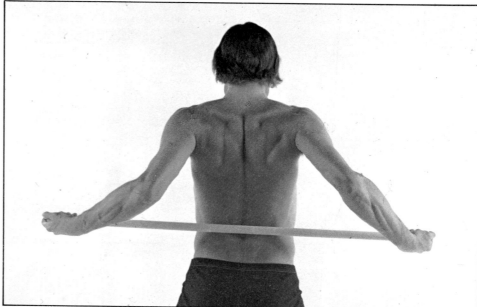

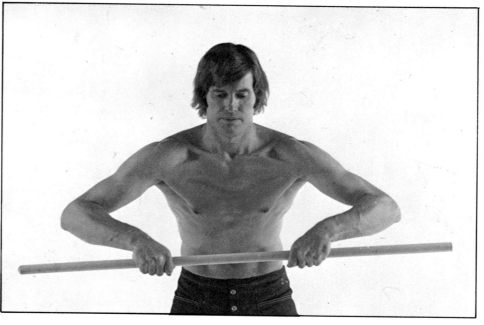

Exercises for Fitness—1

This unique fitness exercise programme has been designed for busy people, people who want to be physically fit and have lithe and supple bodies, but who are unable to put aside the time necessary to become regularly involved in a sport or to visit an exercise class at a set time every day.

These exercises will take you no more than 30 minutes. It is best that you do them every day for several months. After that you can do them three times a week. Although primarily designed for women, they are equally beneficial for men.

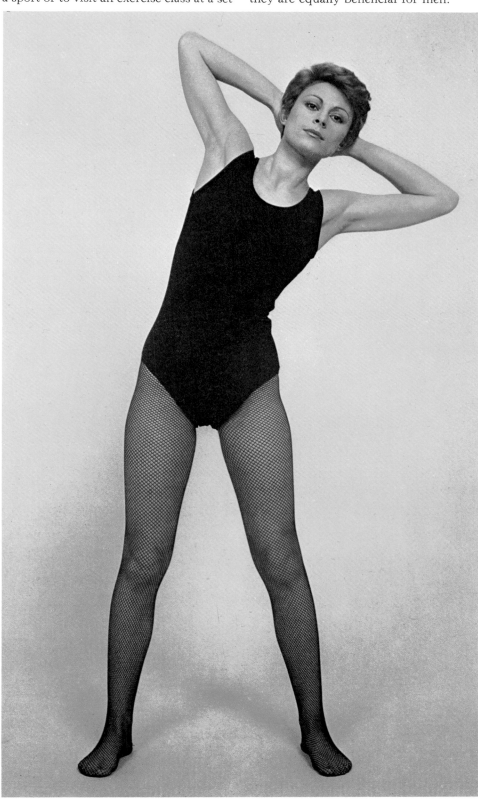

Each part of this course will begin with a series of relaxation and warming-up exercises which *must* be done before every session. They will make your joints more mobile, increase your circulation and loosen up your muscles and ensure that you do not injure yourself during the exercise session.

Every week the warming-up will be followed by seven new exercises, each of which will help to firm and slim a particular part of your body. You'll learn to do exercises which will tone your stomach muscles, firm your breasts, slim your waist, tighten your buttocks and trim your thighs. Do them regularly and you will be delighted with the results.

The first series is quite simple, but the exercises become more difficult as the course progresses and as you become more fit and supple. It is important that you do them in the order given. And if at any time you stop exercising for more than three weeks, you must start at the beginning of the programme and work up again to where you left off.

And, as with any exercise programme, if you have been recently ill, have just had a baby or have a heart condition, check with your doctor before you begin.

Do these exercises at any time of the day that is convenient to you, but always wait for at least one hour after eating. It is best to exercise when you are not tired, but no matter when you do them you will still feel refreshed.

If you find that an exercise is difficult, go only as far as you can and no further. Never strain, and stop immediately if it hurts. You will find after regular and continuous practice that you will become more lithe and what was impossible to do one week requires no effort the next. The first time you do each exercise, look carefully at the photographs as you follow the steps and try to hold your body in the same position as the model. Unless the instructions say otherwise, breathe normally.

Do each exercise only as many times as you can. If you become tired or breathless stop, lie down on the floor and take three deep breaths before continuing. After you have finished each session lie down on the floor and rest for five minutes.

Always wear loose, comfortable clothes when you exercise and be sure to remove all your jewelry.

Remember, if you want to lose *weight* you must diet; if you want to lose *inches* you must exercise. Exercise is the only way to firm your muscles. And for a slimmer, more beautiful figure, a combination of diet and exercise is the most effective way.

Now begin the fitness exercise programme and make it part of your life.

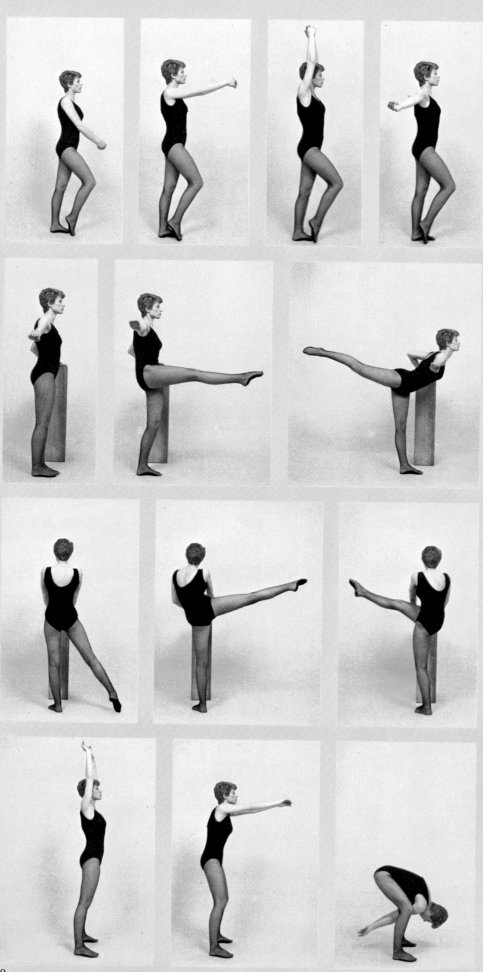

Running on the spot

Stand with your feet together and your arms at your sides. As you circle your arms raise your heels alternately off the ground and "run" on the spot. Do eight steps to each circle of your arms. Between each of the positions shown here, your left leg should bend and your right heel touch the floor. Keep your head up, your shoulders back and your back straight. Repeat 10 times, and increase this by five each day.

Leg swing

Stand next to a chair or any sturdy object which you can hold at chest or waist level. Rest your left hand on the chair and put your right arm out at shoulder level. Keeping your head up, swing your right leg forwards and backwards 20 times, leaning forward when your leg stretches back. Go as high as you can with your leg straight. Turn around and repeat 20 times with your left leg.

Crossover swing

Stand about two feet away from a chair with your hands resting on the top. Extend your right leg to the right as far as possible, and then swing your leg across the front of your body to the left. Keep your legs straight and do not turn your head. Repeat 20 times, then repeat the exercise with your left leg. As with the leg swings, height will come with increased practice.

Through leg swing

Stand with your feet apart. Stretch your arms above your head and, as you bend your legs, slowly swing your arms between your legs and reach back as far as possible. Keep your arms straight. Return to the upright position. Repeat 10 times, and increase this each day by as much as possible without straining or tiring.

58

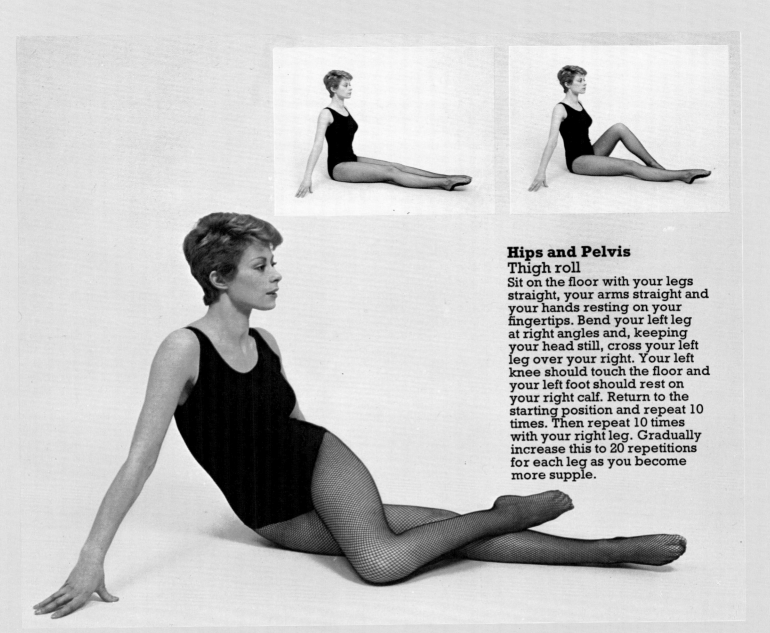

Hips and Pelvis
Thigh roll
Sit on the floor with your legs straight, your arms straight and your hands resting on your fingertips. Bend your left leg at right angles and, keeping your head still, cross your left leg over your right. Your left knee should touch the floor and your left foot should rest on your right calf. Return to the starting position and repeat 10 times. Then repeat 10 times with your right leg. Gradually increase this to 20 repetitions for each leg as you become more supple.

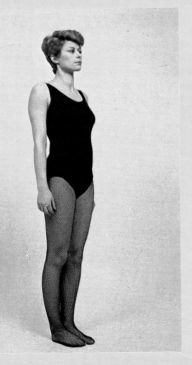

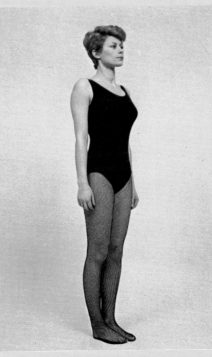

Stomach
Stomach contraction
Stand up straight. Keeping your neck, shoulders and legs relaxed, push out your stomach and hold for a count of one. Contract your abdominal muscles and pull your stomach in as much as possible and hold for a count of two. Repeat 20 times, breathing normally throughout. It is best to do this exercise with your legs slightly bent.

59

Waist
Side bend

Stand with your feet well apart and link your hands behind your head. Keep your back straight. Bend to the right, making sure that your arms are level with your ears, that your elbows are well back, and that your body does not lean forwards or backwards. Return to the starting position, and repeat on your left side. Repeat 10 times, gradually increasing this to 20 repetitions.

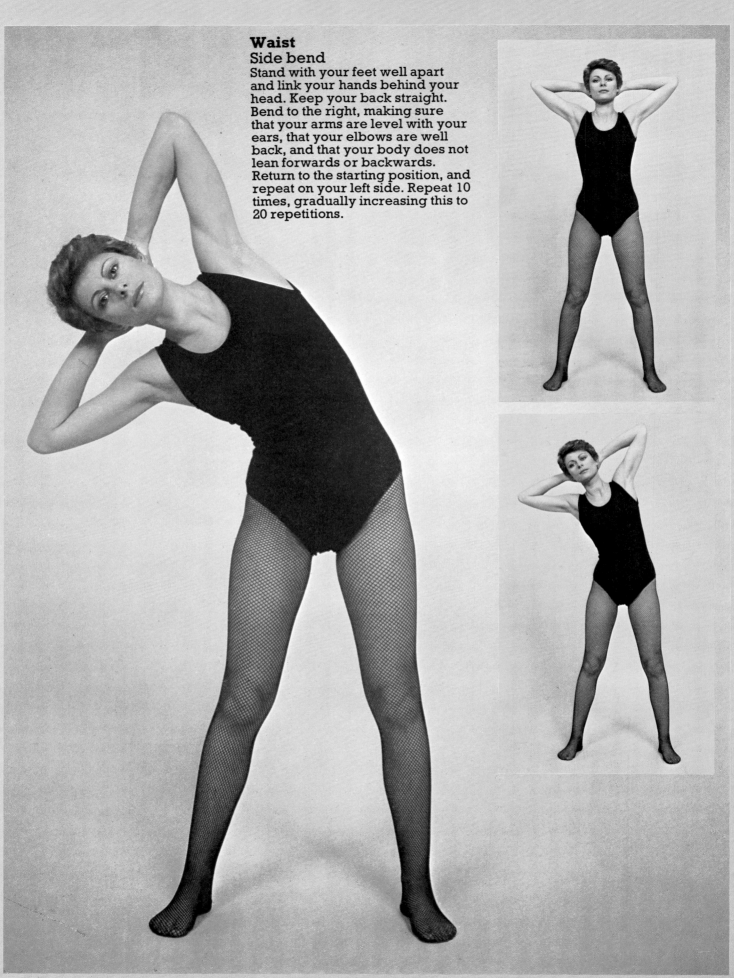

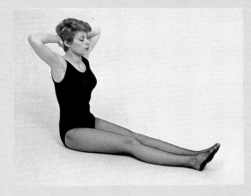
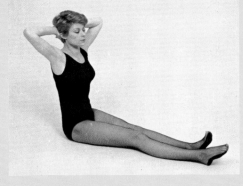
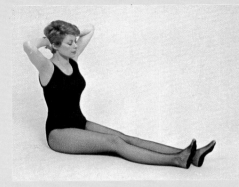

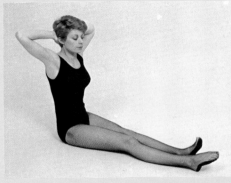
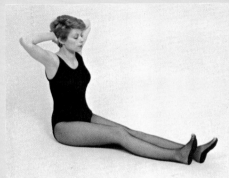

Buttocks
Floor walk
Sit on the floor with your legs straight and your hands linked behind your head. Moving your hips but keeping your head and arms still and your back straight, "walk" forward on your legs and buttocks for 10 "steps". Try not to twist your upper body. Then "walk" back for 10 "steps".

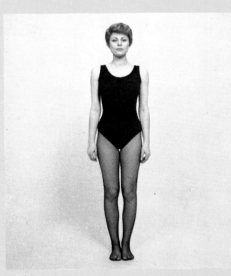
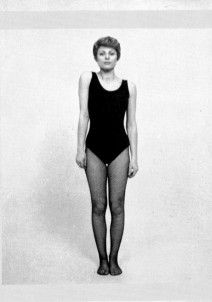
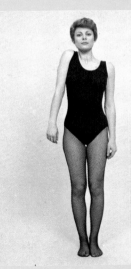

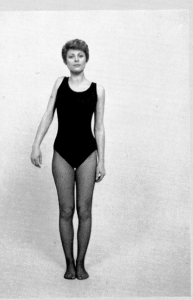
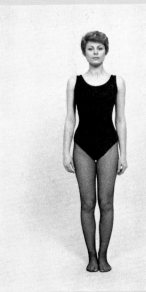

Neck and Shoulders
Shoulder circles
Stand with your feet together and your arms relaxed at your sides. Push your right shoulder forward, lift it up as near to your ear as possible without moving your head, draw it back as far as possible and then return to the starting position. Keep your head still and relaxed throughout the exercise. Do eight circles first with one shoulder and then with the other, then four, then two and finish with one circle with each shoulder.

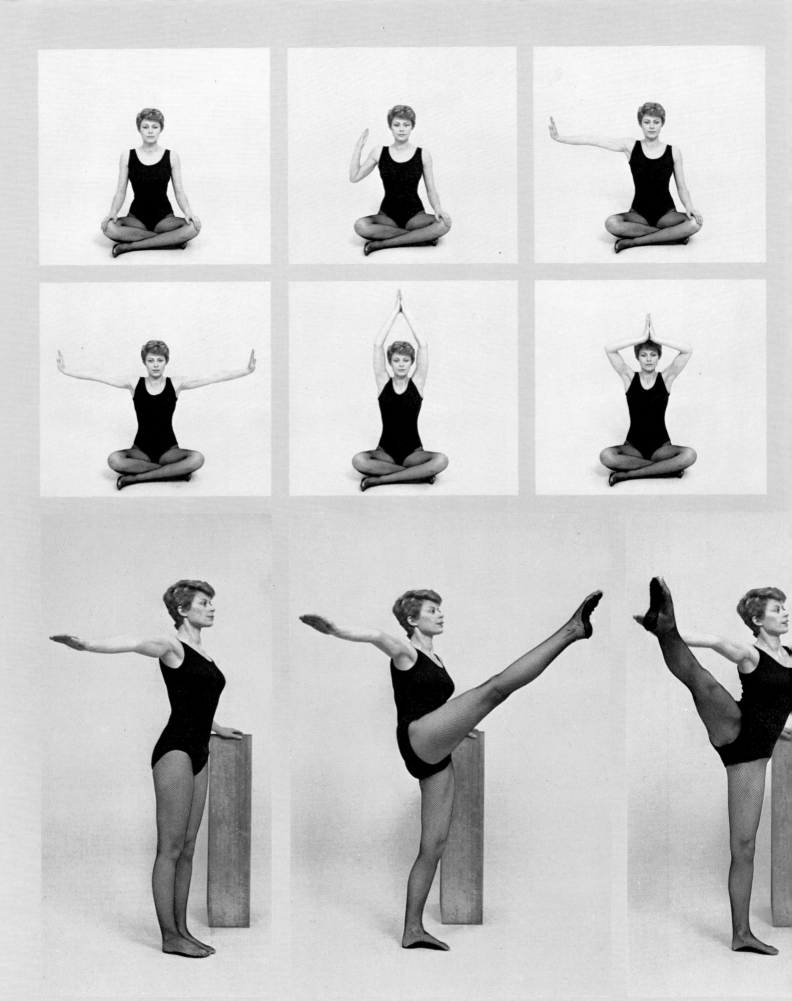

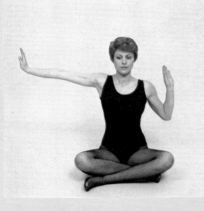

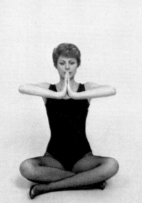

Breasts
Prayer exercise

Sit on the floor with your legs either crossed or out-stretched and well apart. Lift your right hand to your right shoulder, and push slowly out to a count of four, as though you were pressing against a wall. Lift your left hand up and press slowly outwards in the same way. Raise your arms above your head so that your palms are touching. Keeping your elbows well up and pressing in gently, slowly lower your hands to chest level. Then press your hands together hard for a count of six. Repeat once the first time you do this, and repeat once more each day until doing the exercise six times.

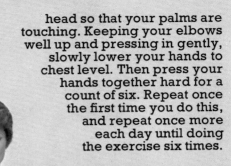

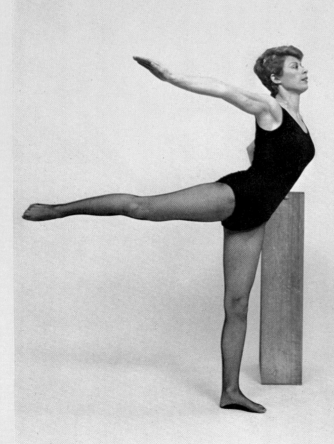

Thighs and Legs
Three-way leg swing

Stand with your feet together. Put your left hand on the top of a chair or sturdy object and stretch your right arm out at shoulder level. Throw your right leg up to the front and bring it back to the starting position. Then push your right leg up and out to the side, and as high as you can. Return to the starting position. Finally, lean slightly forward and push your right leg out behind you, remembering, as with each movement in this exercise, to keep it straight. Try to keep your back straight throughout the exercise. Turn around, put your right hand on the chair and repeat with your left leg. Repeat four times with each leg. You must come back to the starting position between each section of this exercise.

63

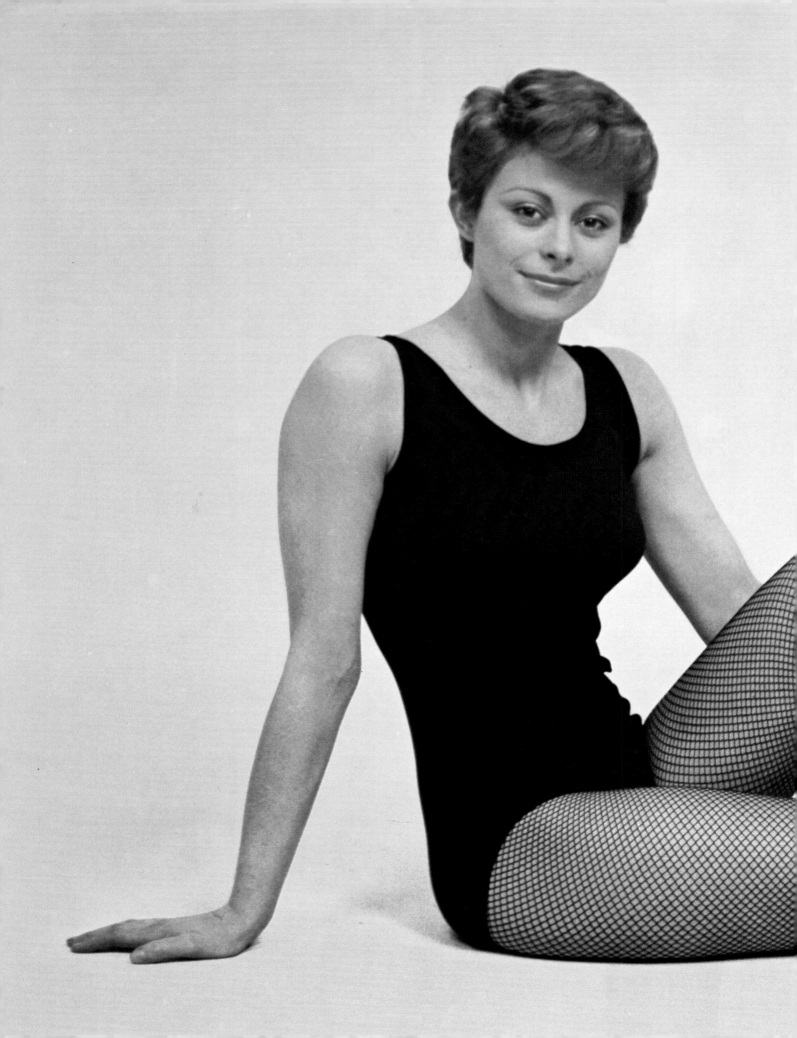

Exercises for Fitness—2

Cut down headaches, backache and nagging pain in the shoulders and arms by learning exercises that relax the neck and shoulders. Physical tension in the neck and shoulders produces aches and pains which in turn, make a person lethargic and irritable. Relaxing the physical tension can ease the mental effects.

It's vitally important to be able to relax this part of your body when you can. But the art of relaxation does not come naturally to most of us; it is something which has to be learned.

The first step is to adopt a sensible overall approach to your body—realizing that it needs care and attention and that it should be respected, but at the same time appreciating that it is your servant. You should be able to recognize which parts of your body are causing tension, and then set about relaxing them.

The next step is good breathing. Most people breathe badly—in short and uneven breaths and too often through the mouth instead of the nose.

Try this simple test. Sit with your head resting on the back of a chair, your feet flat on the floor and your hands in your lap. Make sure that your neck and shoulders are completely relaxed. Now take several deep breaths—really deep ones which fill your lungs to capacity. Inhale and exhale slowly and evenly through your nose. You'll soon find that

With only 30 minutes a day you can be more supple, more relaxed.

this simple action will start to relax your body and calm your nerves. Your tension, both physical and mental, will begin to drain away. This form of relaxation is used throughout the entertainment world, from the theatre to the boxing ring.

Once you have mastered this simple art you'll be able to relax at will—at an office desk, at the wheel of a car, in the cinema. In these situations your brain is no less alert than normal: it is merely that you are learning to control your body more efficiently. And relaxing doesn't mean slouching along with your head forward and your shoulders hunched, or slumping into a chair in a heap at every opportunity. You can hold a good standing or sitting posture without tensing up as long as you know how to relax and breathe properly.

Take a close look at any cat, or when you go to the zoo watch a lion or tiger. They have brought the subject of relaxation to a fine art. A cat can relax because it has complete charge of its body—a body which is remarkably lithe and supple. The next step for you, too, is to cultivate a supple body.

One of the major purposes of this specially designed fitness course is to loosen up the body (all the warming-up exercises do this) and make it really supple. The exercises which relax the neck and shoulders—and which lead to mental relaxation—include the shoulder circles, the head contractions and the head rolls.

This session gives you four warming-up exercises followed by seven new ones —one for each major part of your body.

Do these exercises every day for one week—they take just 30 minutes a day. It's important that you follow the order given, and that you don't strain. If you find one difficult, just do it as best you can. Remember, if you want to lose *weight* you must *diet*; if you want to lose *inches* you must *exercise*. For a slimmer, more beautiful figure you should combine the two.

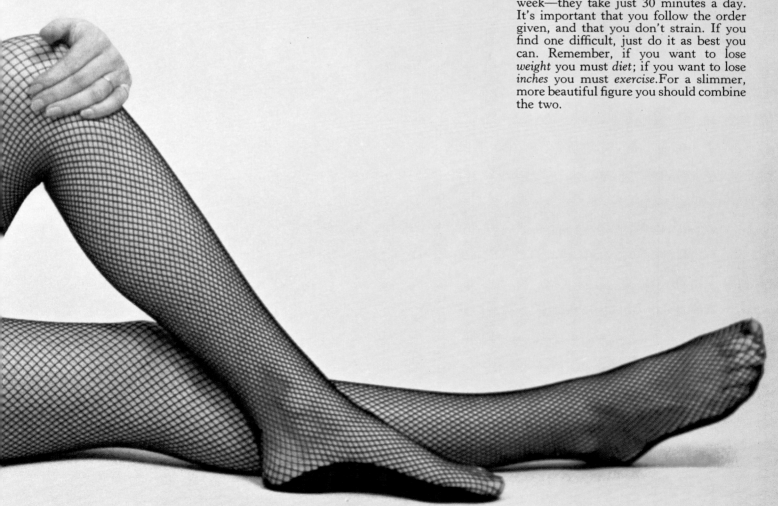

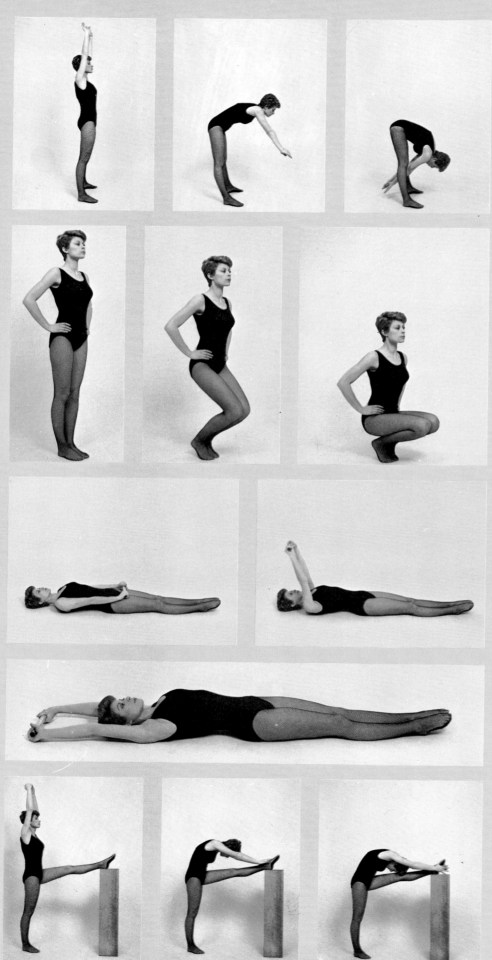

Through leg swing
Stand with your feet well apart and stretch your arms out above your head. Keeping your legs straight, lower your body and swing your arms between your legs. Reach back as far as possible, but keep your arms straight. Repeat 10 times, and increase this by as many as possible each day without feeling tired or strained.
This is a development of the swing in the warm-up for the first programme, where the legs were allowed to bend.

Knee bend
Stand with your feet together and your hands on your hips. Raise your heels and, making sure that your back stays straight and upright, bend your legs and lower your body. If you can, go down as far as your heels, but stop as soon as it strains. Repeat five times.

Overhead stretch
Lie on the floor with your legs straight and your hands resting on your thighs. Hold a light, round, straight object (like a broom handle) in your hands. Breathe in and, keeping your arms straight, bring it over your head until your hands touch the floor. Exhale as you take your hands back to your thighs. Repeat 10 times, gradually increasing this to 20.

Raised leg stretch
Stand about three feet away from a piece of furniture about three feet high. Raise your left leg and rest it on top of the object. Stretch your hands above your head with your fingertips touching. Bend forward, touch your feet with your hands. If you can, touch your knee with your head and link your hands round your left foot.
Repeat twice more, then repeat three times with your right leg. When you have completed the warm-up exercises move on.

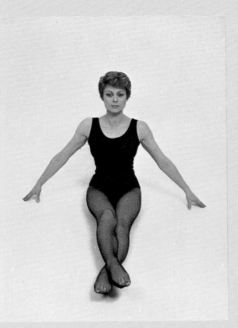

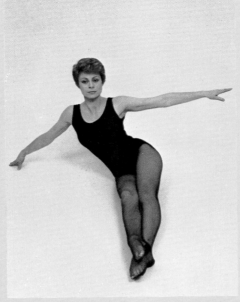

Hips and Pelvis
Hip rock
Sit on the floor with your right leg crossed over your left, your arms out to the sides. Keeping your head straight, rock to the right and your left (main picture). Repeat this 10 times. Come back to the first position, cross your left leg over your right, and repeat 10 times. Increase the number until you do 20 in each position.
Now move on to the stomach exercise.

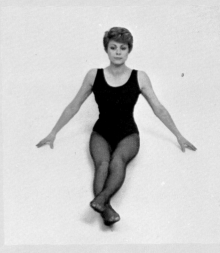

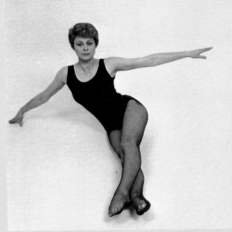

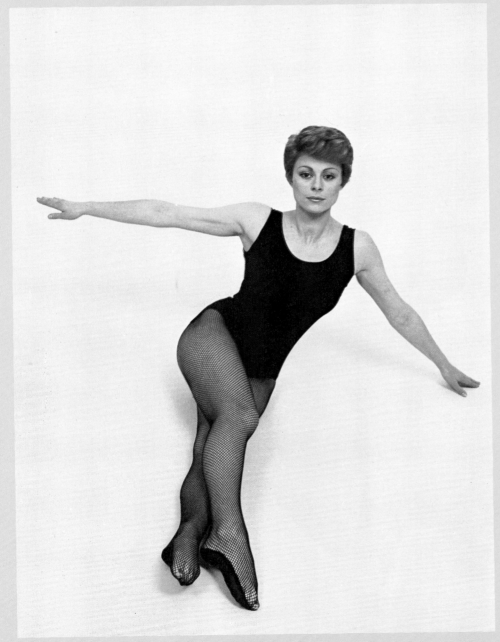

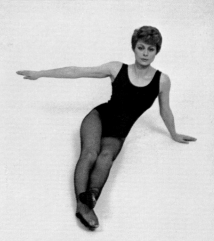

Stomach
Leg raise
Lie on the floor with your legs straight and together and your arms slightly out from your sides, with your palms facing down. Slowly raise your legs to the vertical position. Hold for a count of two, then slowly lower your legs to the floor. Keep your head on the floor throughout the exercise. Repeat five times. When you have been doing this exercise for a few days, do it with your hands linked behind your head.

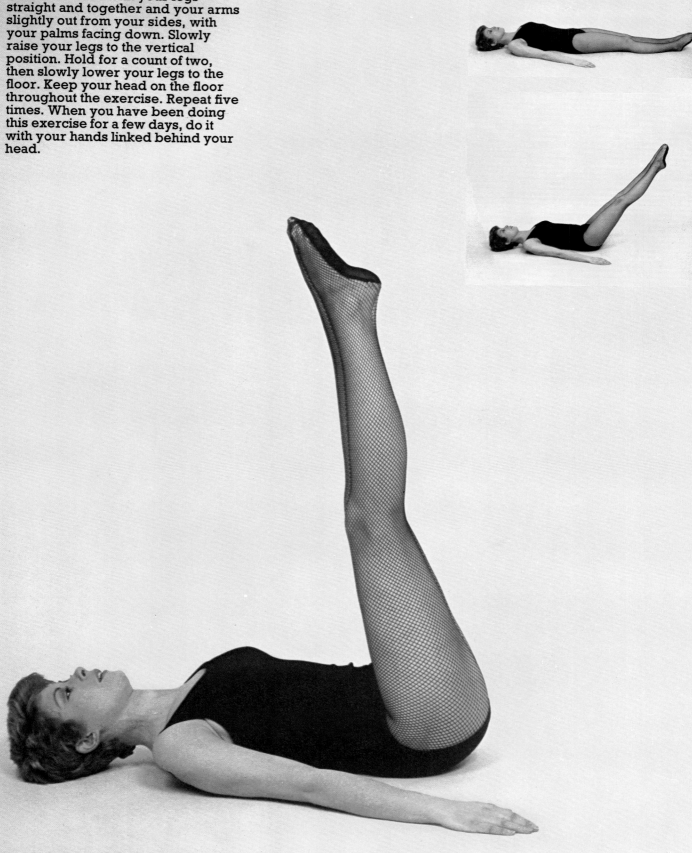

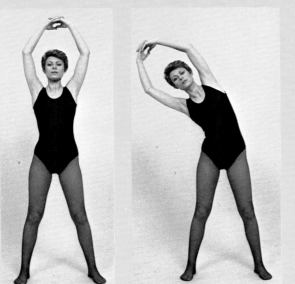
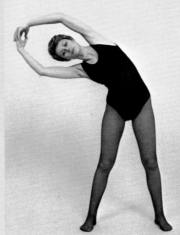

Waist
Side Bend
Stand with your feet well apart and link your hands above your head. Bend slowly to the right as far as possible. Make sure that your arms are held close to your head, that your body does not lean either forward or backward, and that your legs are straight. Return to the starting position and repeat to the left side. Repeat the whole movement 10 times, gradually increasing this to 20.

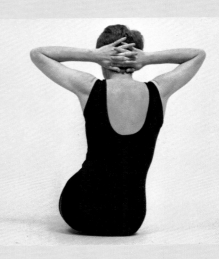

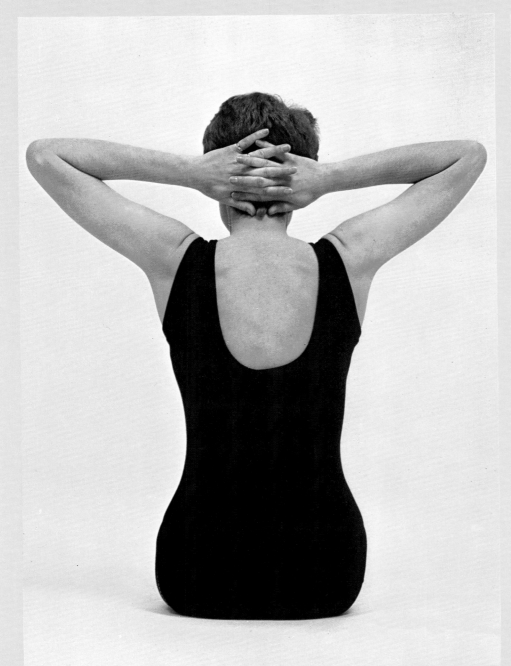

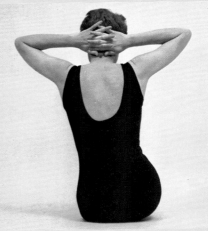

Buttocks
Seated contraction
Sit on the floor with your legs straight and your hands linked behind your head. Contract and then relax first your left buttock to the count of two and then your right buttock to the count of two. Try to keep your body upright. Repeat 10 times, gradually increasing this to 20.
Then go on to the neck and shoulders exercise.

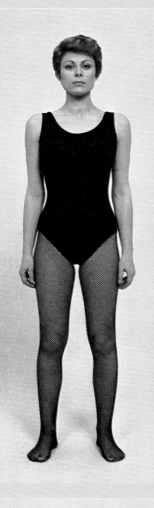
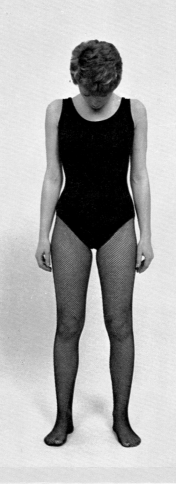
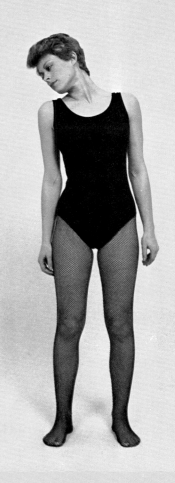
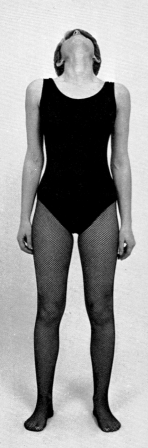
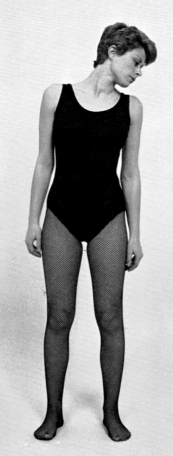

Neck and Shoulders
Head roll

This is one of the exercises that relaxes the neck and shoulder area and relieves mental tension. Stand with your feet slightly apart and your arms at your sides. Keeping your shoulders relaxed and down, drop your head on to your chest. Move your head to the right, keeping your chin close to your shoulder. Roll your head round and drop it back as far as possible. Bring your head round to the left, and then return to the starting position. Repeat the circle, starting by moving your head to the left. The exercise should be done in one smooth movement. Repeat five times.

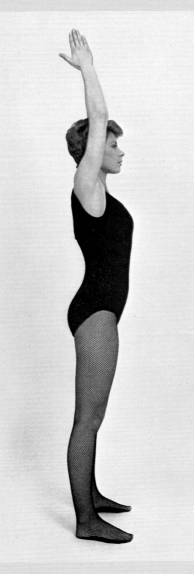

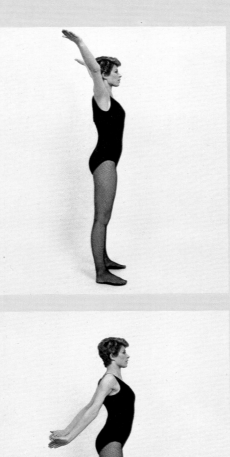

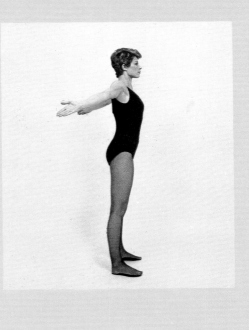

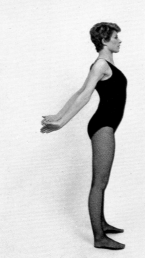

Chest
Diagonal swing
In women this firms the muscles that support the breasts, giving a better bust line. In men, too, this exercise is valuable.

Stand with your feet apart and your hands above your head, then, keeping your arms straight and well back, try to make the backs of your hands touch by swinging your arms diagonally back. Get as close as you can but do not strain. Keep your head up. Return to the starting position and repeat 10 times.

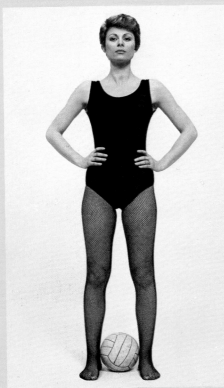

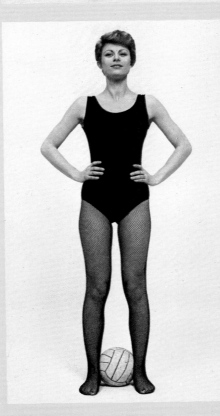

Thighs and Legs
Thigh contraction
Stand with your feet slightly apart and your hands resting on your hips. Contract your inner thigh muscles and try to "pull" your legs together without actually moving your feet or legs. The importance of this exercise is to contract the muscles on the inside of the thighs, and you might find it easier and more beneficial to place an object, such as a hard football, between your ankles.

71

Exercises for Fitness—3

This week's schedule includes two exercises to help your sitting position: the waist swing, which trims your waist and helps you to sit up, and the head contraction, which helps you to hold your head up.

You spend a good deal of your life sitting down—at an office desk, in a car, in the cinema, at the meal table, watching television—and it's vital, both for comfort and the sake of your body, that you try to sit properly.

Don't slump or slouch. The most important factor is to sit with your back straight whenever possible. It doesn't mean you should sit like a ventriloquist's dummy: it is possible to sit well and feel relaxed. With your back straight, you hold your head properly without it poking forward, you keep your shoulders from becoming hunched and give your stomach and diaphragm freedom to function.

Another important factor is that you need adequate support. Make sure your chair is the right height for your office desk; adjust your seat when driving a car for the most comfortable position; don't slump into a soft chair to watch television.

Chairs should be comfortable, practical

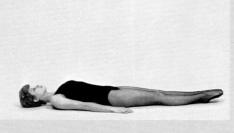

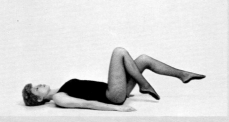

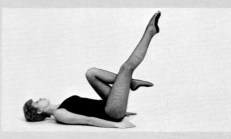

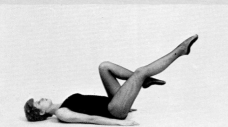

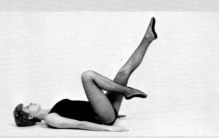

Bicycling
Lie on your back with your arms by your sides and your legs together. Keeping your back flat on the floor, raise your right leg and then your left leg and rotate them, making sure that your knees come up at least level with your hips. Point the toes of your extended leg. Repeat 20 times.

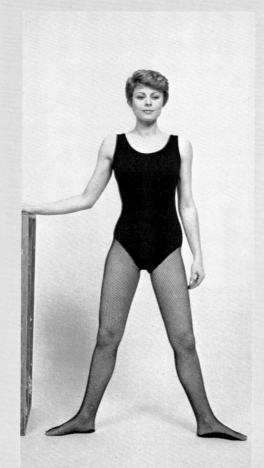

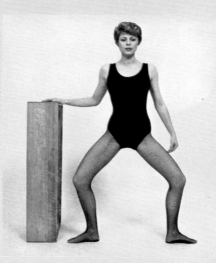

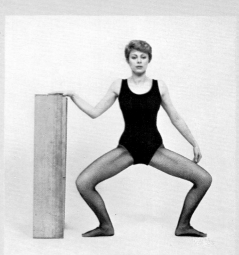

Plie
Stand with your feet apart, a distance of 1½ of your own feet between your heels, your toes out to the side. Rest your right hand on a chair at waist level. Keeping your back straight and upright, bend both knees out over your toes. It is essential that you keep your hips pressed forward and that your knees bend sideways. Lower yourself as far as you can without straining, and then straighten up. Repeat five times, increasing this gradually to 10.

and attractive. For television or reading, your head should be supported; the seat should be firm and deep enough to support the length of your thighs; it should be high enough to allow movement but not to leave your legs dangling.

If you sit badly (though you may well think you are relaxed) the area of your lower spine will become tense. Your muscles become weak, you develop pains in your neck, shoulders and back, and the result is physical tension which in turn can give you headaches and make you irritable. At meal times, too, bad posture means that your body has to work that much harder to digest your food.

This third week of exercises closes the first half of the elementary course. The second half is a little more demanding and more advanced. You should run through the first three schedules before attempting these, working up to maximum repetitions (if you have not already done so) in order to keep fit and supple.

This lesson, like the previous two, is made up of four warming-up exercises followed by seven new ones which you run through in order. It should take you about 30 minutes to complete the course for the third week of exercises.

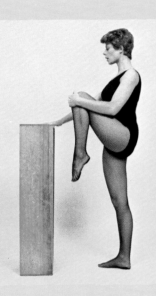
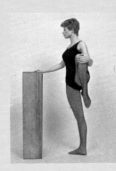
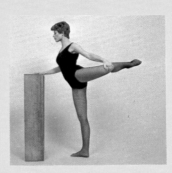
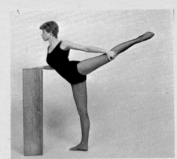

Knee hug
Stand facing a chair with your feet together. Rest your right hand on the top of the chair and bring your left leg up towards your chest, holding your knee and keeping your back straight. Keeping your body still, pull your left leg round to the side and, still holding your knee, pull your left leg back and straighten, taking it as high as possible while leaning slightly forward. Do this exercise to the count of eight. Change round and use right leg. Repeat five times.

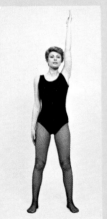
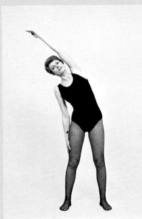
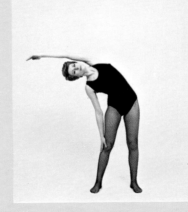

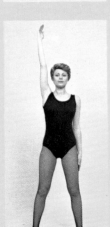
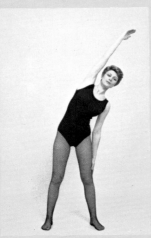
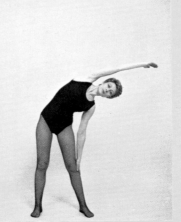

Side bend
Stand with your feet about 18 inches apart and your arms by your sides. Raise your left arm straight above your head. Keeping your right arm straight and your right hand on your leg, give three pulls to your right, bending over as far as you can on the last one. Do not lean forwards or back. Straighten up and repeat five times. Repeat five times with your right arm, bending to your left.

73

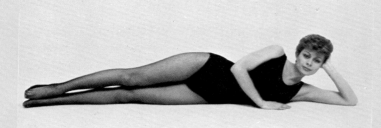

Hips and Pelvis
Side leg raise
Lie on your left side with your left hand supporting your head, your right hand on the floor in front of you and your legs together. Keeping your body still, raise your right leg as high as possible, making sure your body does not lean forward or back. Lower your leg and repeat 10 times. Then turn round and repeat 10 times with your left leg. As with all the exercises, breathe normally unless it says otherwise.

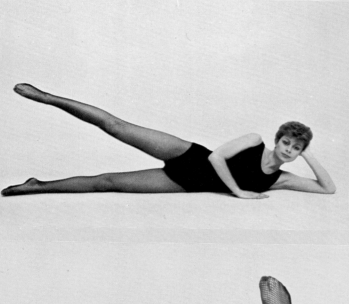

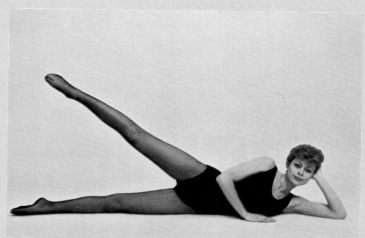

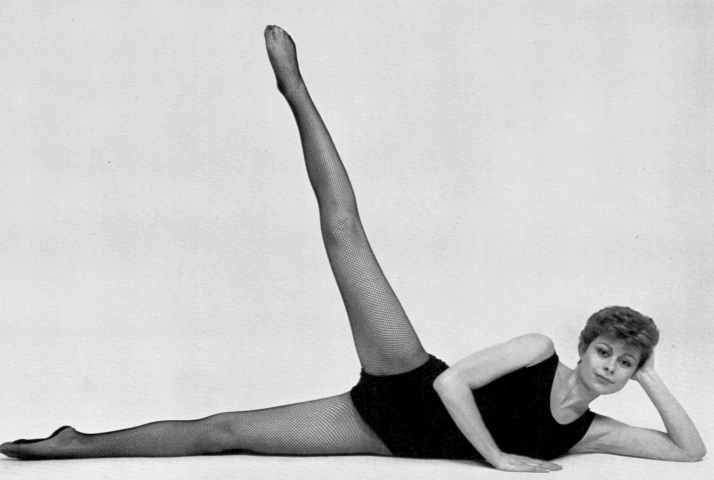

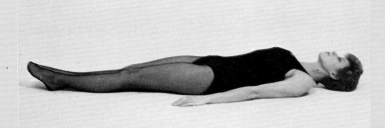

Stomach
Knee to chest raise
Lie on your back with your feet together and your arms by your sides. Keeping your head on the floor, bend your legs and raise your knees to your chest. Slowly extend and then lower your legs and hold at an angle of about 45 degrees for a count of two. Do not lower your legs to the floor. Bend your legs and bring your knees back to your chest. Repeat five times and gradually increase this to 10. Keep your head on the floor throughout the exercise, and do not strain. Now stand up for the waist exercise.

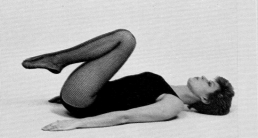

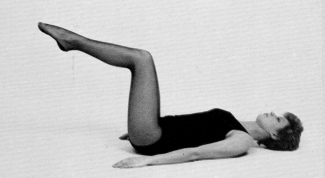

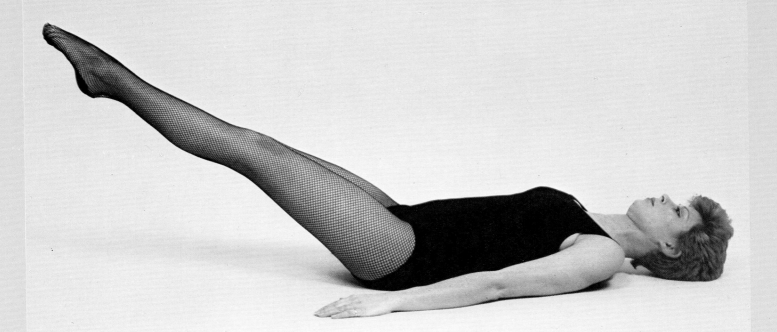

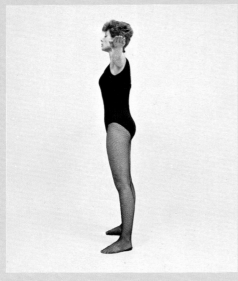

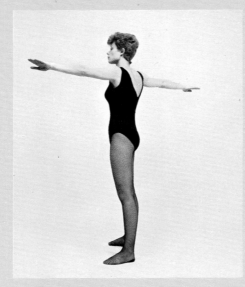

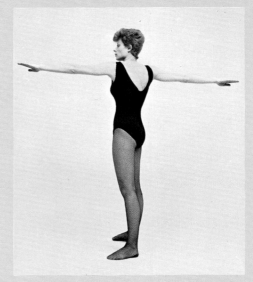

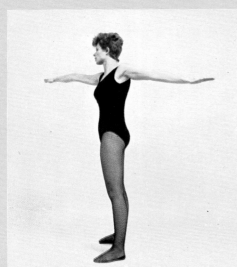

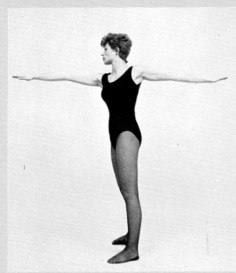

Waist
Waist swings
Stand with your feet about 18 inches apart and your arms to the side at shoulder level. Keeping your arms straight and at the same height, swing your right arm back as far as possible, making sure that your left arm still forms a straight line with it. Swing your left arm round as far as possible to the left, bringing your right arm round to form a straight line. Repeat 20 times, gradually increasing this to 30. Keep your hips still throughout the exercise and remember not to drop the arm that goes back or raise the arm that goes forward.

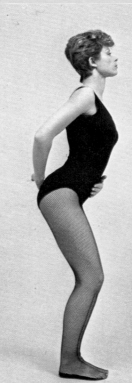

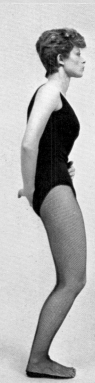

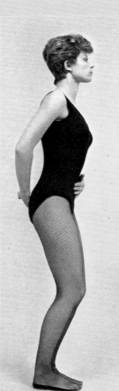

Buttocks
Pelvic contraction
Stand with your feet together and your legs slightly bent. Place the palm of your left hand on your stomach and the back of your right hand on your buttocks. Pull your hips and buttocks back to the count of two, then push your hips forward and tuck your buttocks in to the count of two. Repeat 10 times.

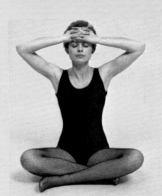 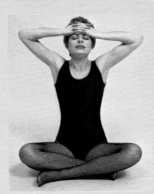 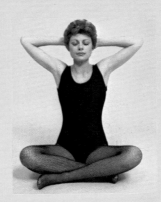

Neck and Shoulders
Head contraction
Sit in a comfortable cross-leg position with your back straight. Link your hands on your forehead, keeping your elbows well up. Inhale and push your hands against your forehead and vice-versa, holding the contraction and the breath for a count of six. Exhale. Link your hands behind your head, inhale, and repeat the contraction, pushing your hands against your head and vice-versa.

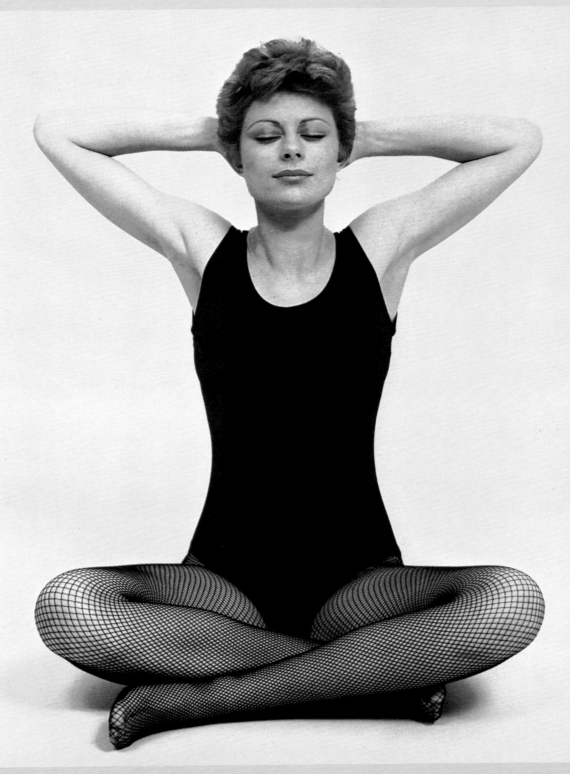

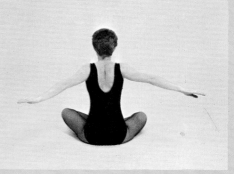

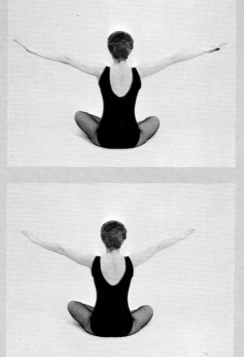

Chest and Breasts
Arm circles
Sit in a comfortable cross-leg position with your back straight and your arms by your sides. Lift your arms to shoulder level. Moving your arms up and backwards, and keeping them straight, make 25 small circles. Repeat in the other direction. Gradually increase this to 50 times in each direction. The arm movement is slightly exaggerated in the pictures to illustrate the effects.

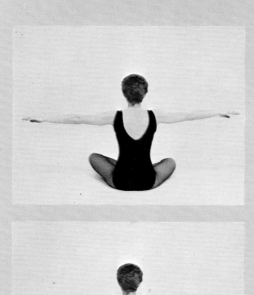

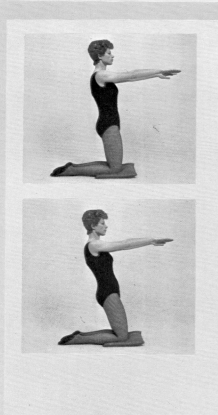

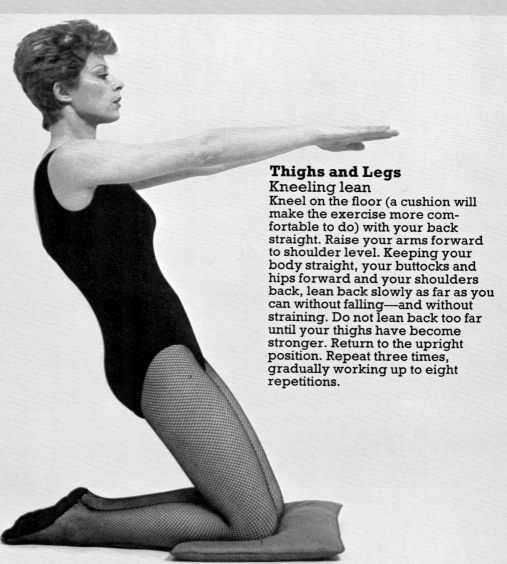

Thighs and Legs
Kneeling lean
Kneel on the floor (a cushion will make the exercise more comfortable to do) with your back straight. Raise your arms forward to shoulder level. Keeping your body straight, your buttocks and hips forward and your shoulders back, lean back slowly as far as you can without falling—and without straining. Do not lean back too far until your thighs have become stronger. Return to the upright position. Repeat three times, gradually working up to eight repetitions.

Exercises for Fitness—4

The Fitness Exercise Course becomes more difficult in this chapter. We've changed the model and we've changed the location to show you can do it all in the comfort and privacy of your own home—but this week's programme is still a natural progression from the third session.

If you've been doing your exercises in all seriousness, working up to maximum repetitions, you'll be quite fit and this week's programme should present no problems for you. If you've let it slip a little—and that's only too easy to do—then resume the course but take it gently. Don't strain, warm up well before you start, and keep to the basic number of repetitions the first time around.

Everyone, of course, must warm up before starting the main exercises. Go through the ones below – the pictures are on page 58 if you need them for reference – and proceed to your 30 minute programme fully prepared. As always, breathe normally unless the instructions say otherwise. Follow any instructions on breathing, to the letter.

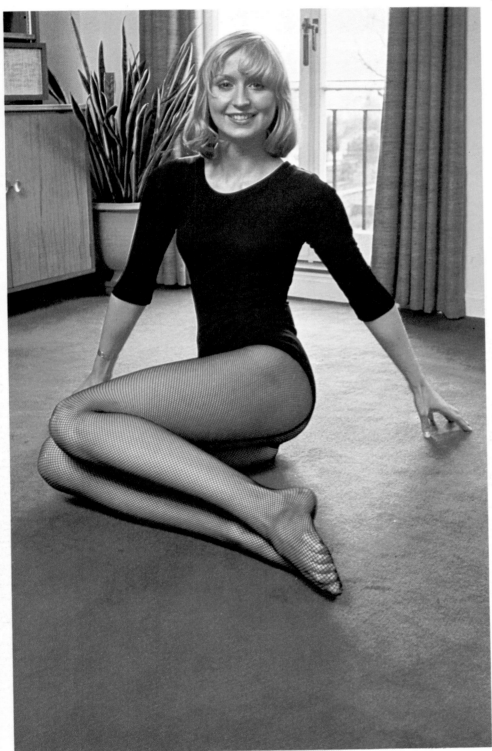

Warm up Exercises

Running on the spot
Stand with your feet together and your arms at your sides. As you circle your arms raise your heels alternately off the ground and "run" on the spot. Do eight steps to each circle of your arms. Between each of the positions shown here, your left leg should bend and your right heel touch the floor. Keep your head up, your shoulders back and your back straight. Repeat 30 times.

Leg swing
Stand next to a chair or any sturdy object which you can hold at chest or waist level. Rest your left hand on the chair and put your right arm out at shoulder level. Keeping your head up, swing your right leg forwards and backwards 20 times, leaning forward when your leg stretches back. Go as high as you can with your leg straight. Turn around and repeat 20 times with your left leg.

Crossover swing
Stand about two feet away from a chair with your hands resting on the top. Extend your right leg to the right as far as possible, and then swing your leg across the front of your body to the left. Keep your legs straight and do not turn your head. Repeat 20 times, then repeat the exercise with your left leg. As with the leg swings, height will come with increased practice.

Through leg swing
Stand with your feet apart. Stretch your arms above your head and, as you bend your legs, slowly swing your arms between your legs and reach back as far asMMM swing your arms between your legs and reach back as far as possible. Keep your arms straight. Return to the upright position. Repeat 30 times.

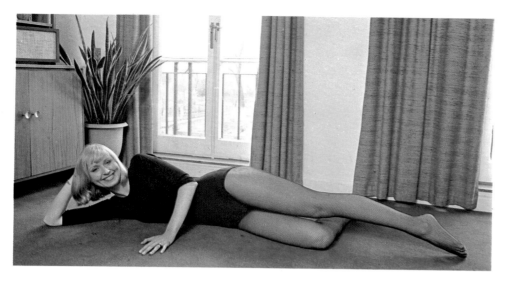

Hips and Pelvis
Side leg raise
Lie on your right side with your head supported by your right hand and your left palm on the floor. Bend your right leg at right angles. Raise your left leg a little and then turn it inwards so that your big toe is touching the floor. Raise your left leg as high as possible, making sure it does not lean forward or back. Then lower to the starting position.
Repeat 10 times, then repeat 10 times lying on your left side and raising your right leg. Gradually increase this to 20.

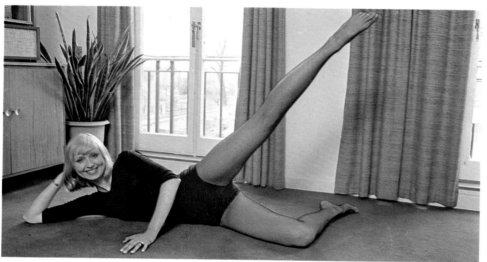

Stomach
The Willow
Stand with your feet slightly apart and your hands linked above your head, your palms facing down. Take your arms behind your head, keeping them straight, and arch your back. Count one, then bring your hands in front of your head and push your pelvis forward. Count two. Try not to bend your legs. Do this eight times, gradually working up to 20 repetitions.

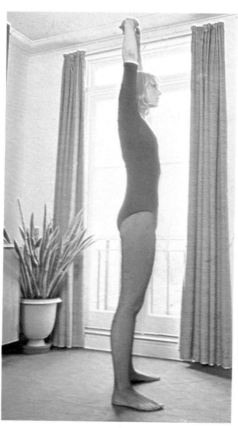
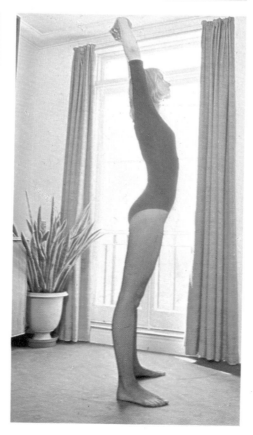
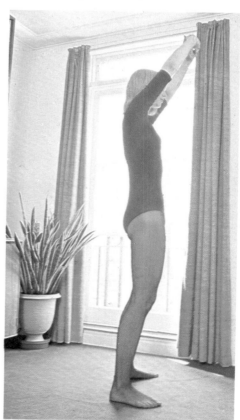

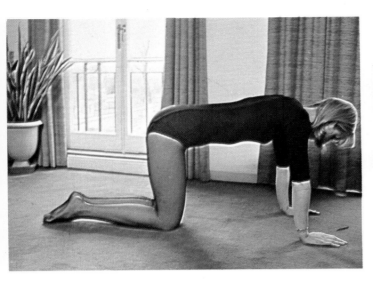

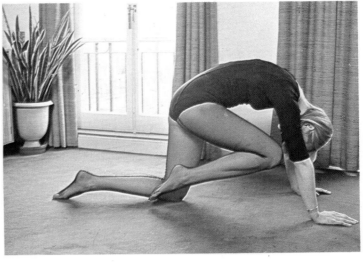

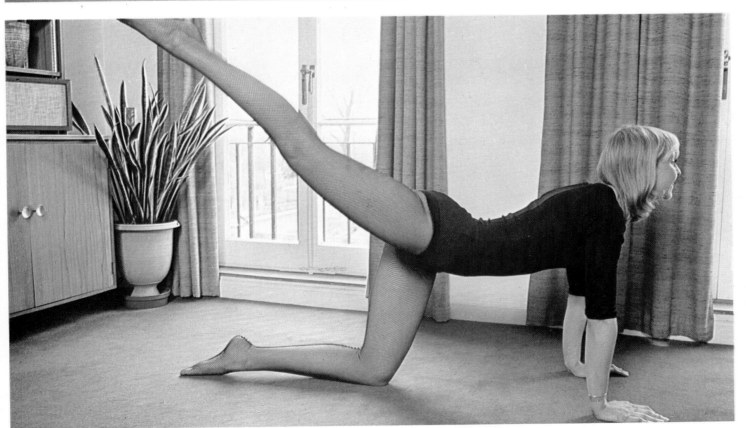

Waist
Bench swings
Kneel on the floor with your hands
below your shoulders. Bend your
right knee up and bring your head
down to touch it. Swing your leg
back until it is parallel to the floor
and look straight ahead, then swing
your right leg up as high as you can
and hold for a count of four.
Repeat 10 times without letting
your foot touch the floor, then 10
times with your left leg. Gradually
increase this to 20.

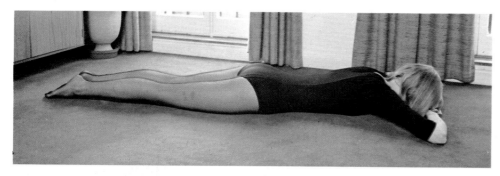

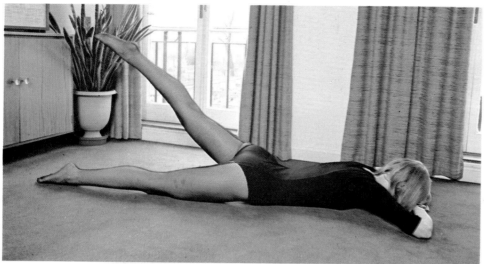

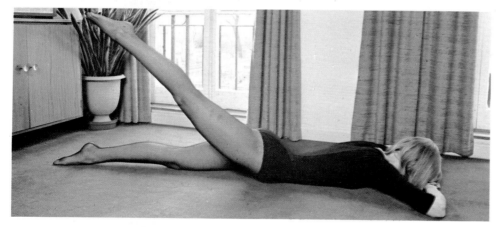

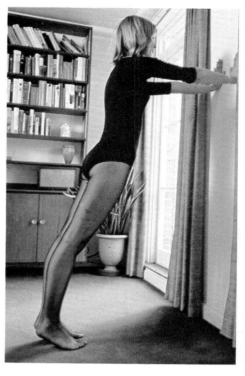

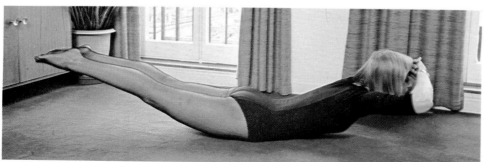

Neck and Shoulders
Wall push
Stand about three feet from a wall with your arms by your sides. Raise your arms to shoulder height with your palms facing the wall. Keeping your body straight, fall towards the wall. Bend your elbows and let your head touch the wall, but do not drop your head. Push yourself away and return to the upright position, leaving your arms in front of you at shoulder height. Repeat 10 times, working up to 20.

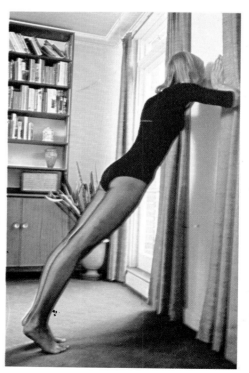

Buttocks
Head and leg lifts
Lie on your front with your legs together and your forehead resting on the backs of your hands. Slowly raise your left leg as far as possible and lower, then raise your right leg and lower. Finally lift both legs and your head, keeping your hands on your forehead and your elbows well up. Hold for a count of four and then lower.
Repeat five times, gradually working up to 10.

Breasts
Arm contraction
Sit in a cross-leg position or stand with your arms crossed, your hands holding your forearms just above your wrists. To the count of 1—2, 1—2, push hard and then pull with both hands.
Repeat 20 times, gradually increasing this to 40.

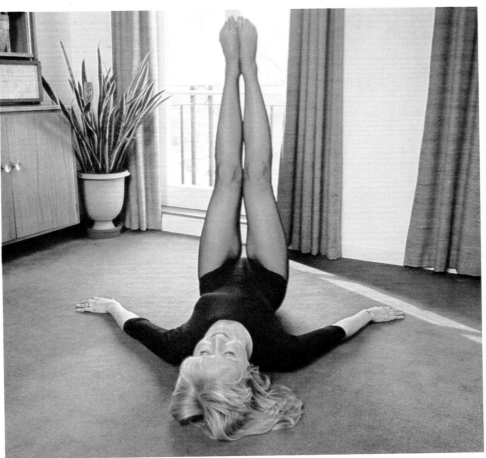

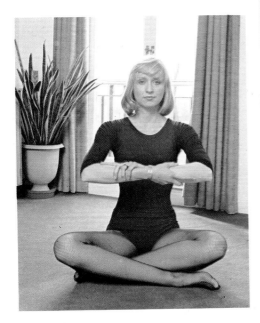

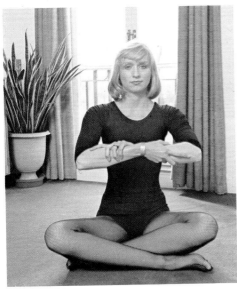

Thighs and Legs
Thigh spread
Lie on the floor with your legs together and your hands on the floor. Raise your legs to the vertical position. Take your legs out to the sides as far as possible, count one, and return to the upright position. Count two.
This exercise should be done rhythmically and vigorously for the best benefits.
Repeat 10 times, gradually working up to 20.

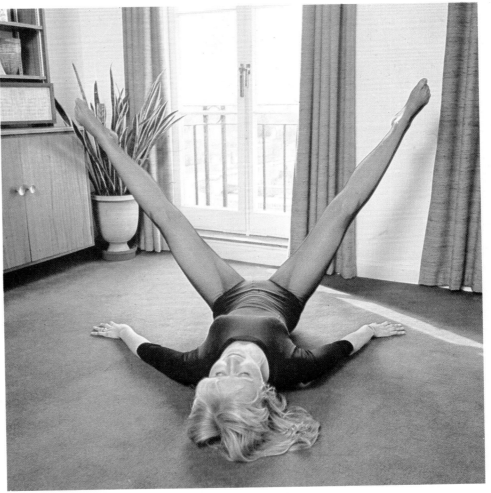

Move well and you'll increase your attractiveness. Walk, stand and sit properly and you'll make an impression whether or not you've got a perfect figure or conventional beauty. All you need is poise.

A woman's walk can be an eye-catching asset in itself. Any woman who 'carries herself well'—head up, shoulders back, ribcage lifted—is going to turn heads.

The Exercise for Fitness Course helps you to stand and move well and makes you more attractive as a result, But, just as important, paying attention to the way you move will help you get the most

from doing the exercises.

If you realize your walking posture is bad, try practising at home with a book on your head, breathing quite deeply.

The same applies to standing. Whether you're at a bus stop, in a shop or at a party, try to think about the way you stand. It's not vanity—it's a sensible approach to gaining and preserving a healthier and more attractive body. And, once you've learned, it will soon become automatic.

Try to keep your weight evenly distributed: putting it all on one leg can damage the hips and cause backache. And avoid leaning forward or back.

If you're on your feet all day—working in a shop or a hairdressers, or teaching, perhaps—don't let fashion ruin your health. Shoes which are too high or too flat, and constricting boots, are damaging over a period of time. And, during your breaks, take the opportunity of putting your feet up to give them a rest.

This is the fifth section of the six-part Exercises for Fitness Course. The warm-up exercises given below should be done before you move on to the main part over the page—whether you've been following the course or not. The whole sequence should take you about 30 minutes.

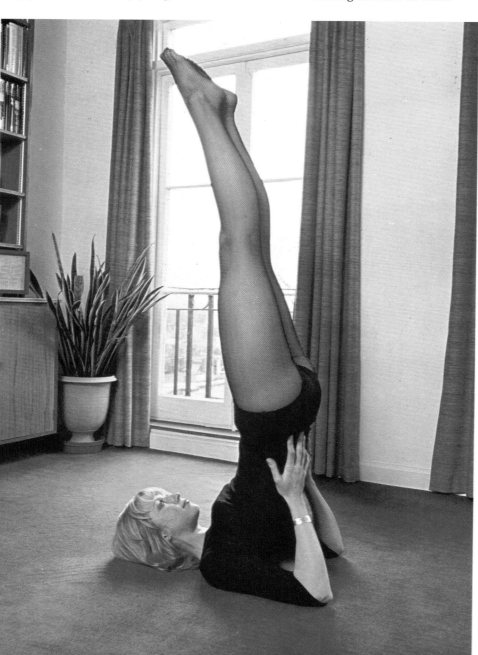

Through leg swing
Stand with your feet well apart and stretch your arms out above your head. Keeping your legs straight, lower your body and swing your arms between your legs. Reach back as far as possible, but keep your arms straight. Repeat 20 times, and increase this by as many as possible each day without feeling tired or strained.

Knee bend
Stand with your feet together and your hands on your hips. Raise your heels and, making sure that your back stays straight and upright, bend your legs and lower your body. If you can, go down as far as your heels, but stop as soon as it strains. Repeat 10 times.

Overhead stretch
Lie on the floor with your legs straight and your hands resting on your thighs. Hold a light, round, straight object (like a broom handle) in your hands. Breathe in and, keeping your arms straight, bring it over your head until your hands touch the floor. Exhale as you take your hands back to your thighs. Repeat 20 times, gradually increasing this to 30.

Raised leg stretch
Stand about three feet away from a piece of furniture about three feet high. Raise your left leg and rest it on top of the object. Stretch your hands above your head with your fingertips touching. Bend forward, touch your feet with your hands. If you can, touch your knee with your head and link your hands round your left foot.
Repeat four times, then repeat four times with your right leg.

Hips and Pelvis
Leg scissors
Lie on your right side with your
legs together, your head resting on
your right hand and your left hand
on the floor in front of you.
Keeping your legs straight, lift
them off the floor and move them
back and forth in a scissor
movement parallel to the floor.
A wide, slow action is easier, a
quick, short action is harder.
Do this for as long as you can,
working progressively up to 40
movements.

Stomach
Sit up bicycling
Lie on your back with your legs
together and your arms out to the
side. Bend your knees, raise your
right leg and bicycle four times. On
the fifth extension of your leg sit
up and take your hands off the floor,
balancing on your buttocks.
Continue bicycling to the count of
four and, on the fifth extension, lie
back on the floor but continue
cycling with your legs.
Repeat the exercise five times.
When your stomach muscles
become stronger you should be
able to do this exercise with your
hands behind your head.

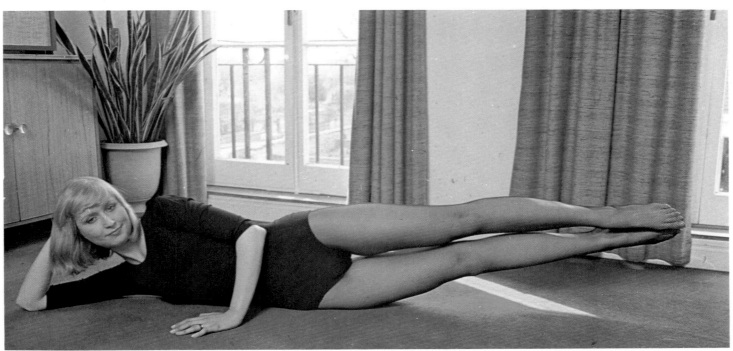

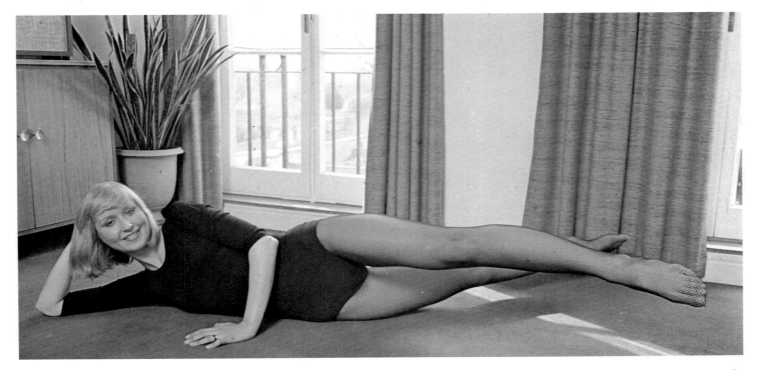

85

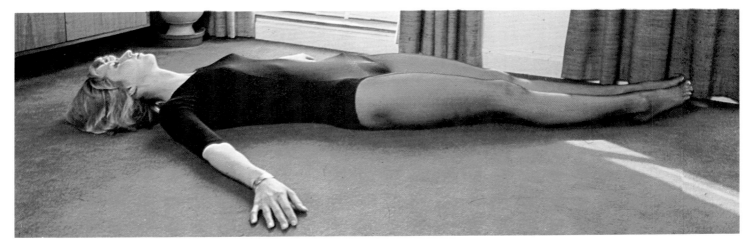

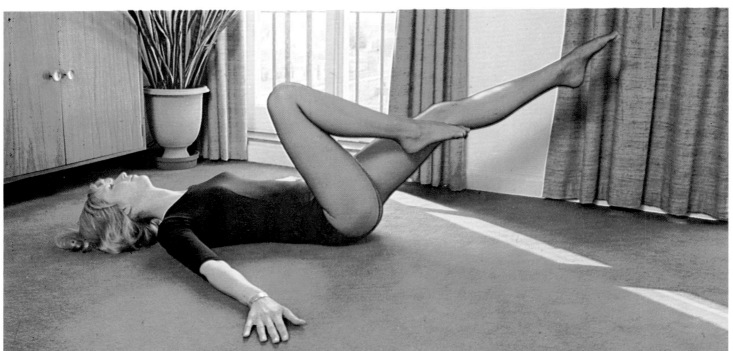

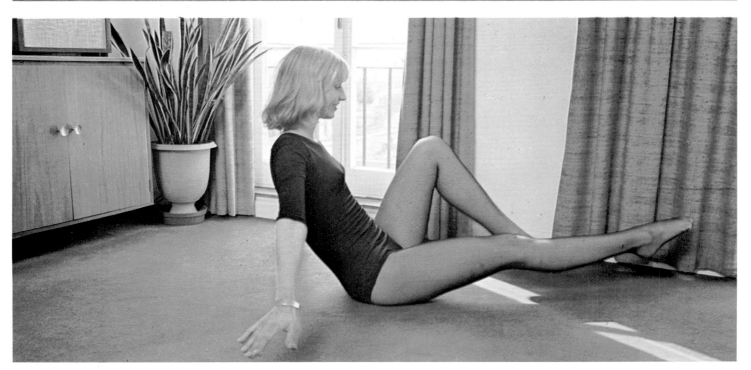

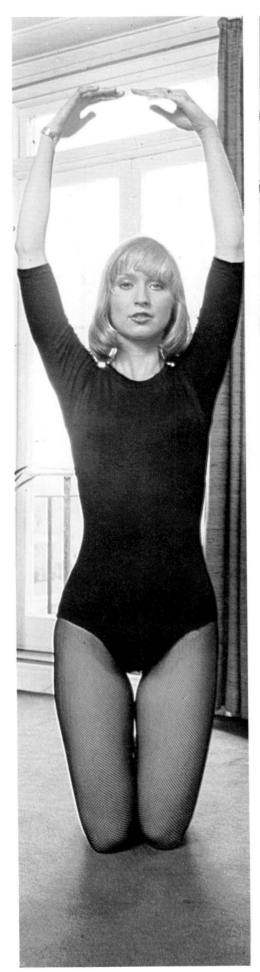

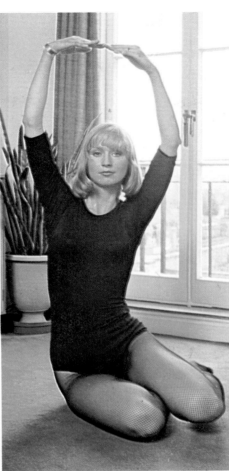

Buttocks
The Mermaid
Kneel up with your body straight
and your arms above your head.
Keeping your body facing forward
and your arms still, lower your
buttocks to the floor on your right
side. Return to the upright position
and lower to your left side.
Repeat five times to each side,
gradually increasing this to 10.

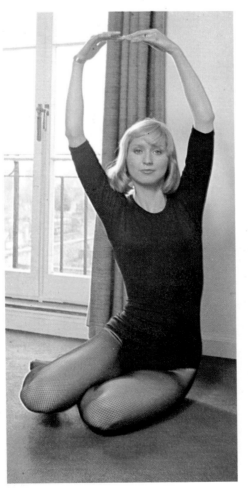

Waist
Body stretch in rotation
Stand with your feet slightly apart
and your arms above your head,
your hands turned inwards.
Keeping your hips facing forward,
turn your upper body to the right
and stretch out as far as you can.
With your arms over your head,
lower your arms and body round in
a circle to your feet and then
continue up to your left, stretching
out as far as you can. Try to keep
your hips still throughout the
exercise. Return to the upright
position.
Repeat four times to your right,
then four times in the opposite
direction.

87

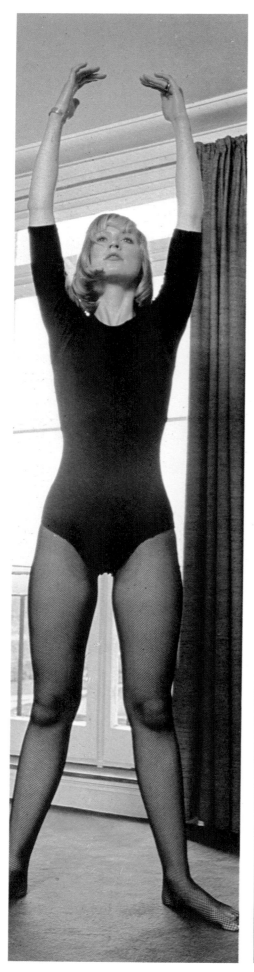

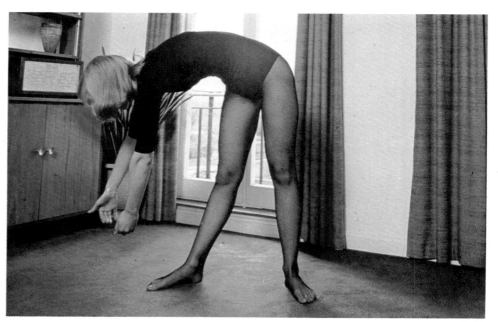

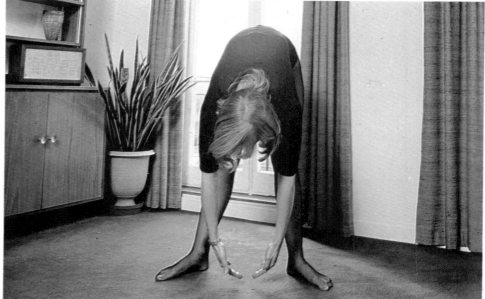

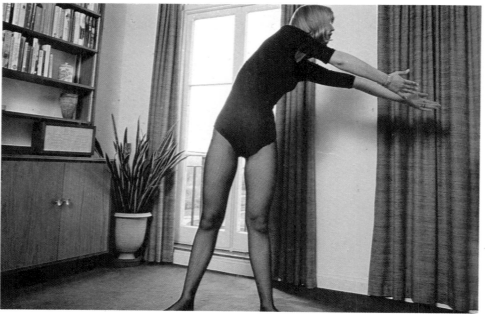

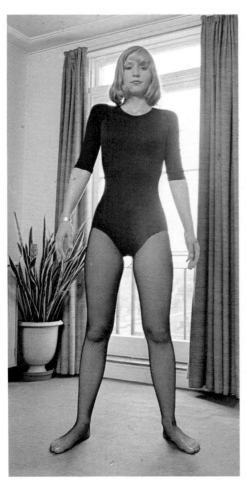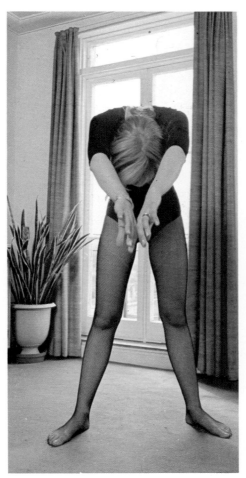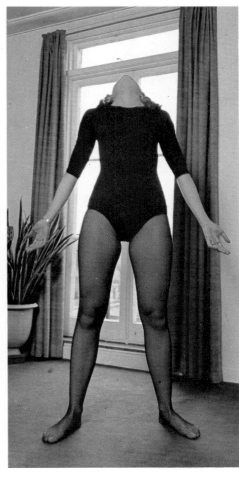

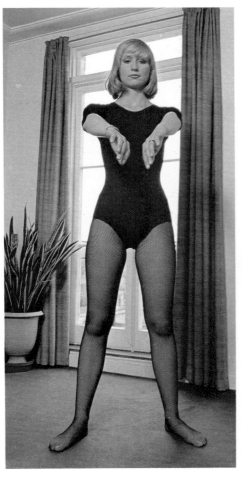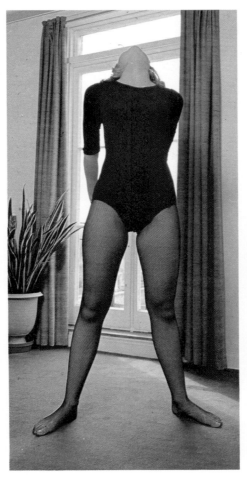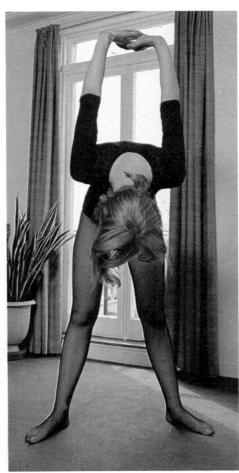

Neck and Shoulders
Arm and shoulder raise
Stand with your feet slightly
apart and your arms by your sides.
Raise your shoulders up towards
your ears. Then, raise your arms to
shoulder level with the backs of
your hands touching. Drop your
head and shoulders and count to
four. Raise your shoulders again
and drop your head back, bringing
your arms out to the sides with
your palms facing up. Hold for a
count of four.
Repeat the whole exercise five
times.

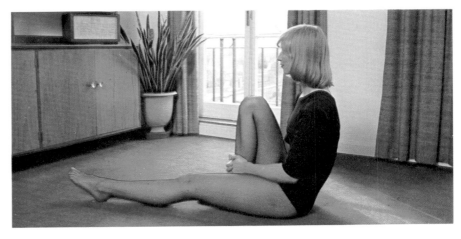

Breasts
Firm breasts—1
Stand with your feet slightly apart
and your arms by your sides.
Breathe in and take your arms
forward, touching the backs of your
hands together. Take your arms
back and link your hands behind
your back, palms up. Breathe out,
then lean back and drop your head
for a count of two. Come up and lean
forward, breathing in. Hold for a
count of two, then breathe in. Do not
lean past waist level, but try to get
your arms as upright as you can.
Repeat twice.

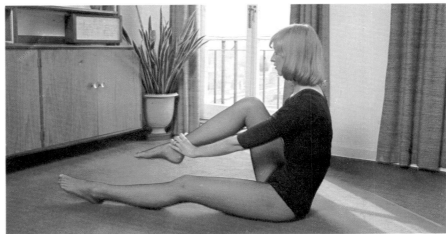

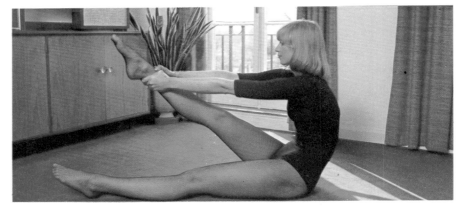

Thighs and Legs
Complete stretch
Sit on the floor. With your left leg
straight, bend your right knee and
clasp the front of your right ankle
with both hands, bringing your
right heel to your buttocks. Keeping
your hands on your ankle, point
your right foot and straighten your
right leg. Pull your leg up as high as
possible and, if you can, touch your
knee with your head. Try to keep
your back straight. Hold for a count
of two. Point your foot again, and
lower your leg to the floor.
Repeat twice with your right leg,
then repeat the whole sequence
with your left leg.

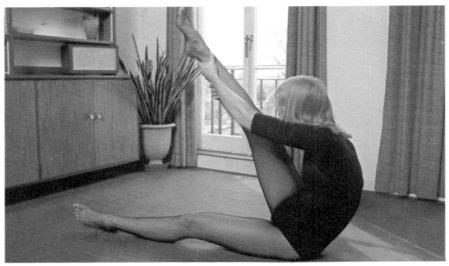

Exercises for Fitness—6

The Exercises for Fitness Course is a continuing programme. You choose just how you want it to develop and how long you want to carry on. You can go on repeating the six parts in turn, gradually building up to maximum repetitions; or you may feel one particular lesson did you more good than the others; or you may prefer to concentrate on one area of your body (such as your breasts or hips) and continue with the relevant exercises.

The overall intention of the course is to help you become more fit, more healthy, more attractive. But there are other benefits. Your balance will improve, your posture will be better, your enjoyment of life can be greater. Above all, perhaps, you'll feel more relaxed.

Relax—it does you good
Most of us don't relax often enough—or in the right way. We think we're relaxing as we watch television, or read, or lie in the sun. But are we?

It's best if you do nothing when you relax. Just lie on your back and try to let your mind go blank. If you're very tired, it will help to put your feet on a cushion, a bed, or even a chair.

Relaxation is an art, and it needs practice. If you really try you'll soon find you can blot out all your problems and worries for a while.

And, once you've mastered it, you'll be able to use your ability to renew your energies. You'll be able to get off to sleep more quickly, and then enjoy a better night's rest as a result. Become conscious of every part of your body, thinking about each in turn from the toes to the head and relaxing one after the other. You'll probably fall asleep by the time you're halfway up.

As always, start with the warm-up programme (the pictures are on page 72 if you need them for reference) and breathe normally unless the instructions state otherwise.

Bicycling
Lie on your back with your arms by your sides and your legs together. Keeping your back flat on the floor, raise your right leg and then your left leg and rotate them, making sure that your knees come up at least level with your hips. Point the toes of your extended leg. Repeat 30 times.

Plie
Stand with your feet apart, a distance of $1\frac{1}{2}$ of your own feet between your heels, your toes out to the side. Rest your right hand on a chair at waist level. Keeping your back straight and upright, bend both knees out over your toes. It is essential that you keep your hips pressed forward and that your knees bend sideways. Lower yourself as far as you can without straining, and then straighten up. Repeat 10 times, increasing this gradually to 20.

Knee Hug
Stand facing a chair with your feet together. Rest your right hand on the top of the chair and bring your left leg up towards your chest, holding your knee and keeping your back straight. Keeping your body still, pull your left leg round to the side and, still holding your knee, pull your left leg back and straighten, taking it as high as possible while leaning slightly forward. Do this exercise to the count of eight. Change round and use right leg. Repeat 5 times.

Side bend
Stand with your feet about 18 inches apart and your arms by your sides. Raise your left arm straight above your head. Keeping your right arm straight and your right hand on your leg, give three pulls to your right, bending over as far as you can on the last one. Do not lean forwards or back. Straighten up and repeat 10 times. Repeat 10 times with your right arm, bending to your left.

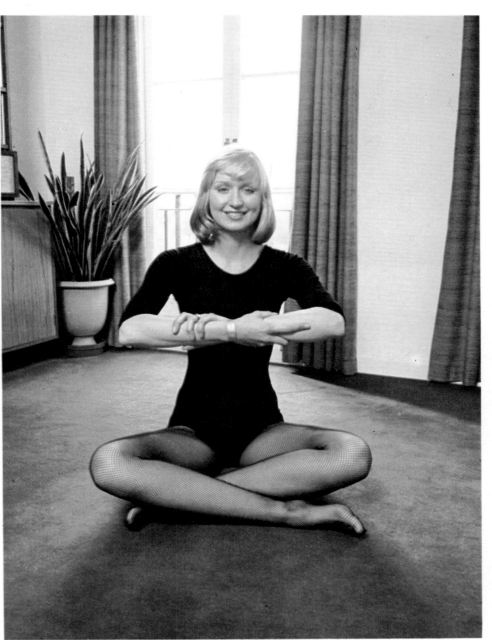

Hips and Pelvis
The Triangle

Lie on your back with your legs
straight, your arms out to the side
and your palms on the floor.
Breathe in and lift your legs up to
the vertical position. Count one,
two, then breathe out and swing
them over to the right until they
touch the floor. Keep your head,
shoulders and arms on the floor.
Count one, two, then breathe in and
bring your legs back to the vertical
position. Count one, two, then
breathe out and swing your legs
over to the left. Count one, two,
then breathe in and return to the
vertical position. Count one, two,
then breathe out and lower your
legs to the floor.
Repeat the whole sequence four
times, gradually increasing this to 8.

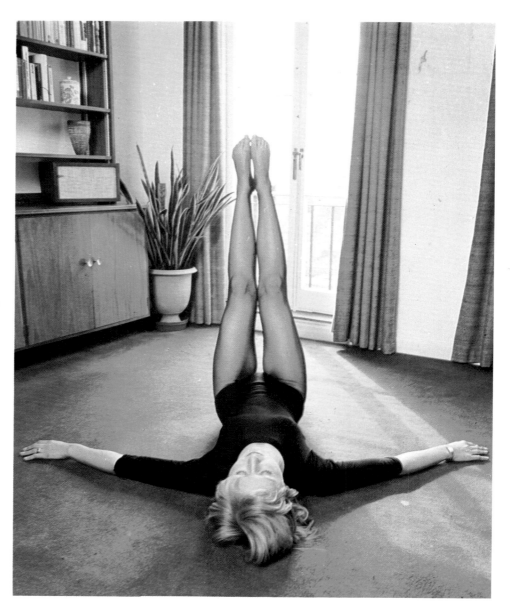

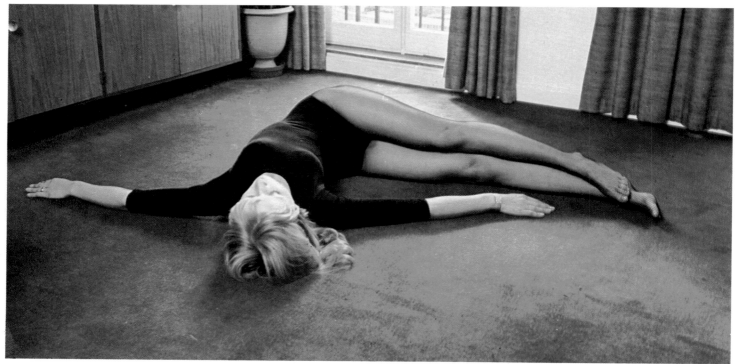

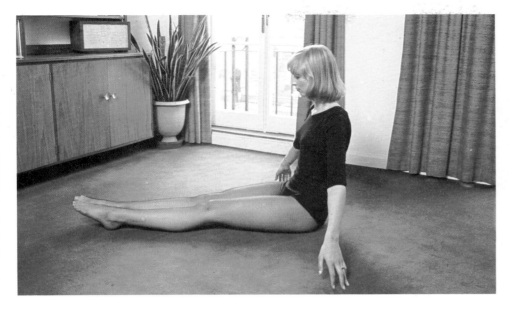

The Stomach
The Seal

Sit up with your legs straight and your arms out to the side, your fingertips touching the floor. Leaning back, raise your arms and legs, making sure that your legs are straight and together. Then open and shut your legs in short sharp movements, like a seal with its flippers.

Start with five movements and increase this by as much as possible each time as your stomach muscles become stronger.

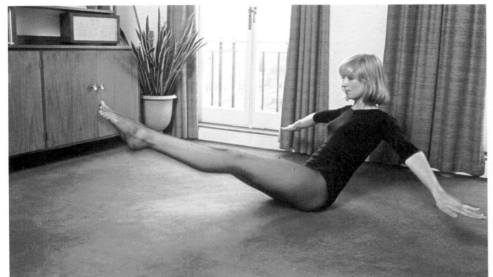

Shoulderstand and leg extension

This exercise, which increases circulation, improves the suppleness of the spine and stimulates the thyroid gland, is an ideal 'bonus' that you can do at the end of your normal programme.

Lie on your back with your arms by your sides. Push down with your palms and slowly raise your legs to hip level. Swing your legs back and support your hips with your hands. Slowly straighten up and hold for a count of eight.

Your body and legs should be in a straight line, your body forming a right-angle with your head.

Come down gently, bending your knees and lowering your legs so that your knees are close to your head. Place your hands back on the floor and roll forward slowly, keeping your legs straight upwards, then lower them. When they touch the floor, let your body go limp and relax.
Repeat twice.

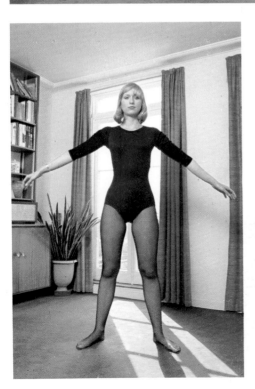

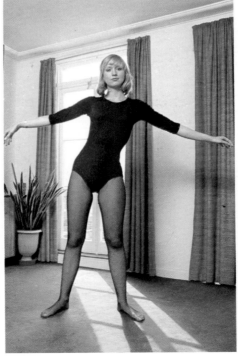

Waist
Ribcage shift

Stand with your feet apart and your arms out to the side. Keeping your hips still, lift up your ribcage and place it over to your left side. Lift up again, return to the starting position, and then repeat to your right side. Try not to strain and do not hunch your shoulders. Practising in front of a mirror will help you to see whether you are doing the exercise correctly.
Repeat 10 times, gradually working up to 20.

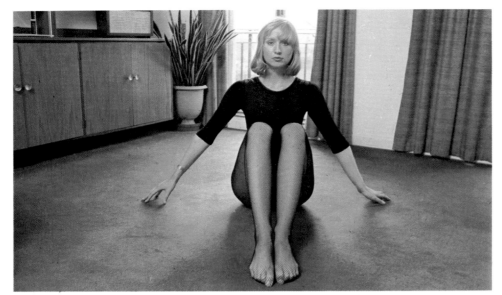

Buttocks
Hip and thigh bounce
Sit on the floor with your knees bent and your arms out to the side, your hands slightly behind you. Keeping your knees together, move them over to the right and 'bounce' them on the floor. Count one, then swing your knees over to the floor on the left side, count two. Try to keep an even, rhythmic movement. Repeat 10 times, counting one, two each time your legs touch the floor, and gradually increase this to 20 times.

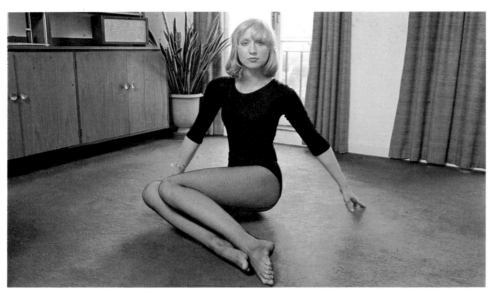

Neck and Shoulders
Standing arm raise
Stand with your feet apart and, with your arms straight, link your hands behind your back with the palms facing each other. Keeping your legs straight, bend forward from the waist and pull your arms up as high as possible. Get your head as near to your knees as you can without straining.
Lower your arms, stand up again, and repeat the exercise five times.

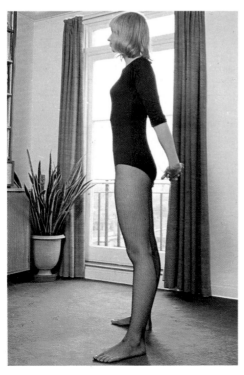
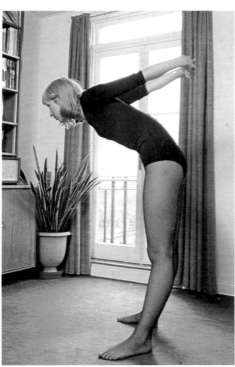
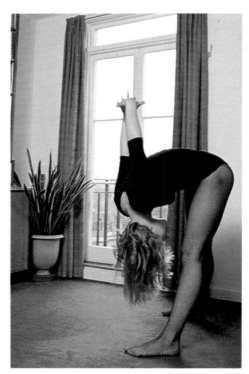

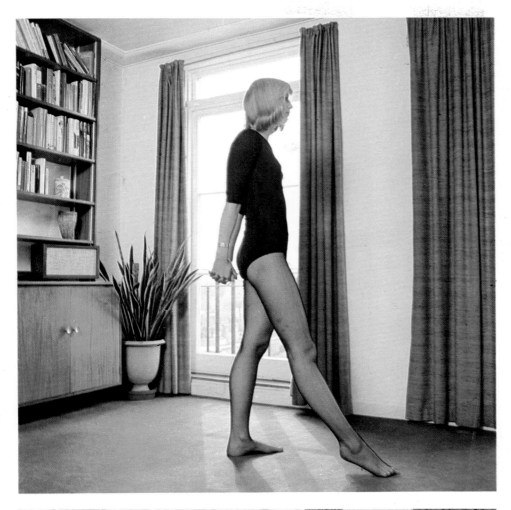

Breasts
Firm breasts—2
First, repeat the exercise for breasts in section five of this course : standing with your feet slightly apart, take your arms forward with the backs of your hands touching. Take your arms back and link your hands behind your back, palms together. Lean back and drop your head for a count of two. Come up and lean forward, lifting your arms up at the back as far as possible. Hold for a count of two.

Now come up and lower your arms. Extend your right leg and, keeping your left leg straight, lean down to touch your right knee with your head, taking your arms up as high as possible. Repeat twice, then repeat with your left leg extended.

> If you've been following this course, and have felt it doing you good, then continue with your exercises.
>
> This six-part programme is intended as a basic guide : you can carry on repeating the sections, you can pick out the exercises you most enjoyed or the ones which did you most good. You won't get too tired of them.
>
> You can incorporate the Streamline exercises, a light weight training programme or a routine of energetic exercises for the more ambitious.

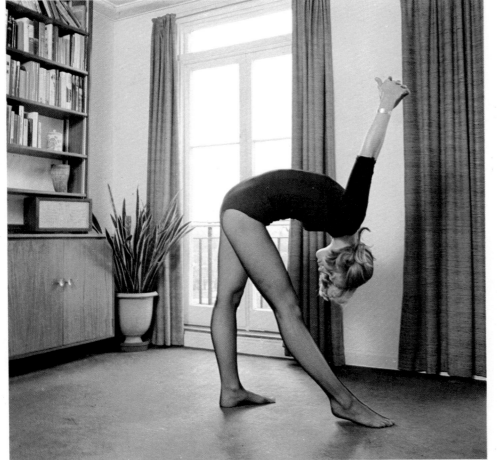

Thighs and Legs
Advanced bench swing
Kneel on the floor with your hands directly below your shoulders and your knees in line with your hips. Bend your left knee off the floor and take your head down to touch it. Swing your left leg back as far as possible and arch your back. With your leg well up, lower your body by bending your arms until your chest and head are on the floor. Return to the starting position and repeat the exercise with your right leg.

Repeat four times with each leg, gradually working up to 16.

95

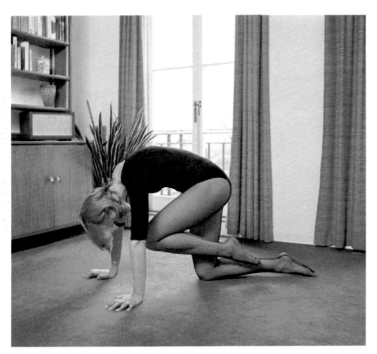
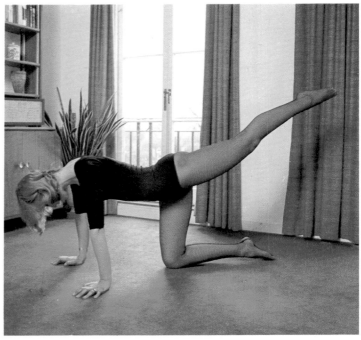
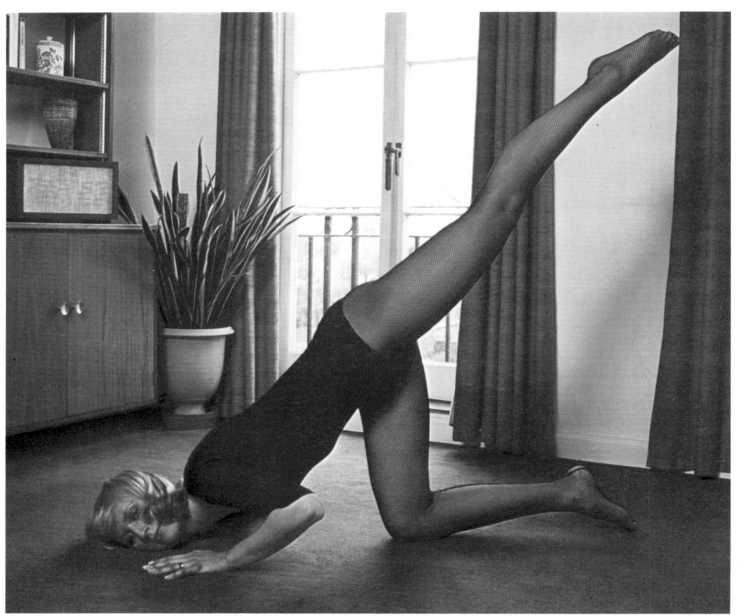

Keep your hands supple

Exercise 1
Hold a pencil on the palm of your left hand with the palm of your right hand. Roll the pencil up and over the finger tips of your left hand and down the back to the wrist without dropping it.
Repeat three times.
Change hands and repeat.

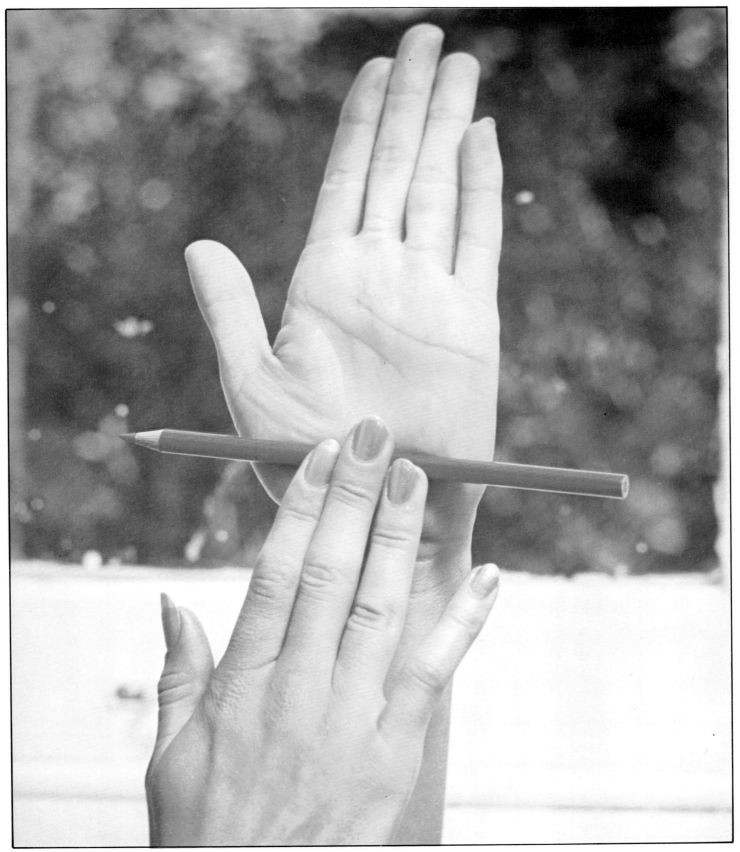

WRIST STRENGTHENING

Exercise 1
Place the palms of your hands together, elbows apart as if you were about to pray. Now, pressing hands hard together, throw them forwards in a rapid jerky movement. Then bring them back to the vertical position again. Keep palms together throughout the movement. Repeat.

Exercise 2
With arms outstretched rotate wrists slowly in a clockwise movement, then repeat in the other direction.

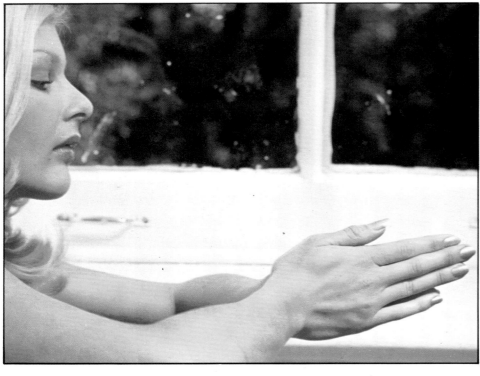

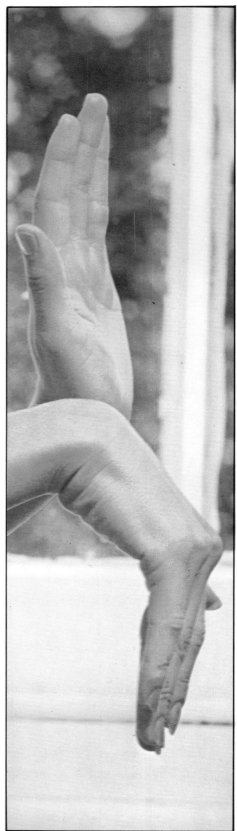

FINGER MOBILITY

Exercise 1
Hold a pencil between the thumb and first finger of your left hand. Now, without using your right hand twist the pencil between each finger, then back again. Repeat once, then repeat with your right hand.

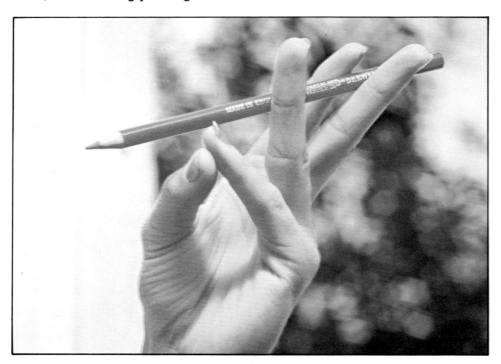

Keep Your Face Fit-1

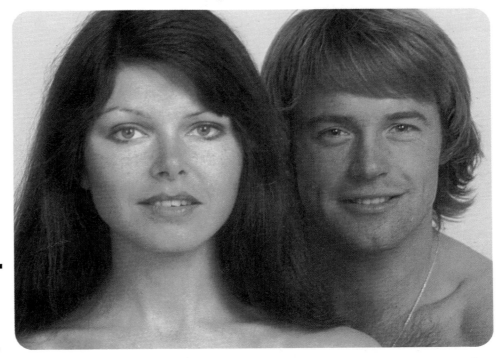

Your face is part of your anatomy—and much more. It can convey all your real or feigned emotions—happiness, sadness, wonder, fear, disgust, anger. It can also conceal your feelings. Some people believe that facial expression reveals a great deal about characters.

The appearance of your face is basically determined by the structure of your bones. But your expressions are created by the action of the muscles.

The true facial muscle lies in thin sheets between bone and skin. This kind of muscle, which is not found anywhere else in the human body, is not uncommon among other mammals.

There are 14 major facial muscle groups. They have one main anatomical function—to open and close the "holes" in the face—the eyes, nostrils and mouth. But these muscles also affect the way a person looks.

After adolescence the skin begins to dry out and becomes less elastic, and the facial muscles start to lose their strength. In time, the combined effects of expression lines and muscular action etch themselves on to the face. Someone who frowns all the time will probably have premature and pronounced wrinkles—long lines across the forehead and little vertical grooves between the eyebrows. And while a lined face can have great character, it can also make a person look old and bad-tempered.

It is not difficult to maintain and improve the tone of the facial muscles and skin. Diet, adequate rest and relaxation play an important part. A body which is well nourished, but not over-fed, and a smooth, firm face usually go together. Fatigue can make your face haggard—the muscles of the face, like all muscles, grow slack with tiredness.

Your state of mind, too, plays a vital part in the way you look. A face which is mobile reflects an active mind and is more attractive than a face which lacks animation. A happy face looks younger than a dejected one. And sadness, depression and worry may cause facial muscles to sag.

When you catch sight of your reflection in a mirror or a shop window and you see a drooping mouth and a furrowed brow, make a conscious effort to look cheerful. Whenever you notice that you are frowning or feel that your mouth is tense and set in a hard line, try to relax the tight muscles. Let your forehead relax and lift the corners of your mouth—you can see and feel the effect immediately.

And just as exercise prevents the muscles of the body from becoming flabby or can restore their tone, there are a number of facial exercises, which should be done by men as well as women, which will strengthen the muscles of the mouth, jaw, neck, cheeks, forehead and around the eyes.

The sooner you begin the better.

Young people in their twenties often develop expression lines and wrinkles but this, as well as the aging process, can be retarded if the facial muscles are kept firm.

Facial exercises do not, of course, work miracles. After middle age they cannot be expected to produce the effect of a surgical face-lift. But they will help at any age. With facial exercises as with any other exercise, the activity stimulates the circulation and as a result the skin looks fresher.

When you do facial exercises always sit comfortably upright on a straight chair. Practice, at first, in front of a mirror. Then, when you have learned the movements and feel confident that you are doing them correctly, you can, if you prefer, do them without a mirror whenever you have a few free moments during the day.

The exercises need not all be done at once. Do as many different ones as you have time for, concentrating on those which you think will do most for your own face. Do not strain or do any exercise which feels uncomfortable. As your facial muscles grow stronger increase the number of times you repeat each exercise.

You may think that you look silly grimacing in front of a mirror, but remember that you are moulding a firmer, smoother and more attractive face.

FACIAL EXERCISES

The facial exercises which follow are the first part of a three part course which has been specially designed to help you to keep your face fit and to look healthier, younger and more attractive. And they will help you to relax when you are feeling tense and over-tired.

When you're tired, look in the mirror and see what gravity does to your mouth. The weary, slackened muscles allow the corners to droop and your whole expression takes on an air of dejection. Exercise will strengthen the muscles around your mouth and help to prevent this sagging, or to correct it when it occurs. Exercise is also a good defence against a double chin and heavy jowls.

The course begins with an exercise for the whole face and a series of exercises for the mouth and jaw. Make these exercises a part of your daily routine.

Whole Face

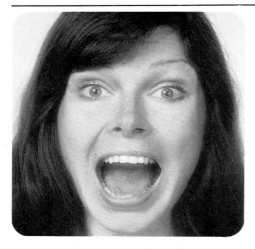

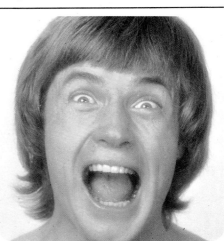

Stimulates the circulation and releases tension using all of the muscles of the face
Abandon your inhibitions for this exercise

Open your mouth and eyes as wide as you can, stretching your face as much as you can.

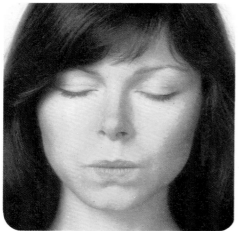

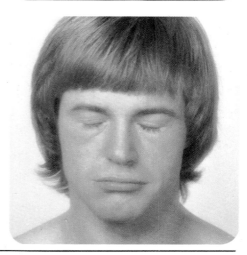

Now close your eyes and mouth and tighten your whole face as much as possible.
Do this whole exercise three times.

Mouth and Jaw

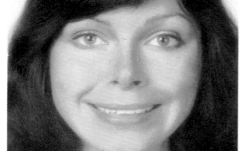

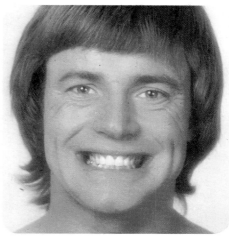

1
Strengthens the jaw and throat muscles, keeps the mouth firm and lips smooth

Say EEX in an exaggerated way.

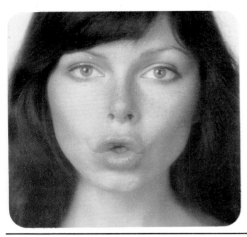 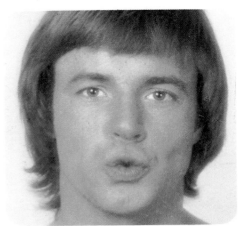

Immediately afterwards say CUE.
Say EEX and CUE 20 times in rapid
succession.

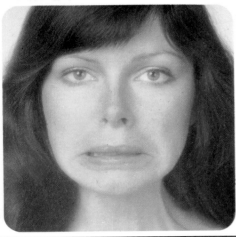 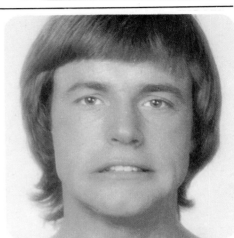

2

**Firms the jaw line and helps to
strengthen the muscles at the
front of the neck**

Stretch the corners of your mouth
down and outwards, keeping your
upper lip as still as you can. You
will feel your throat muscles contract.
Do this 20 times.

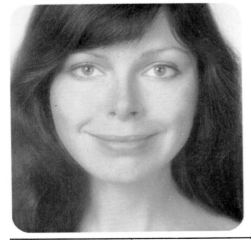 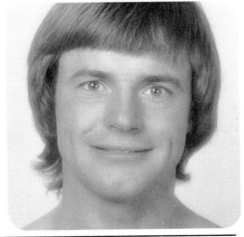

3

**Strengthens neck muscles, firms
the jaw line and works on the
nose-to-mouth lines**

Raise the corners of your mouth in
an artificial smile, keeping your
upper lip still.
Do this 20 times.

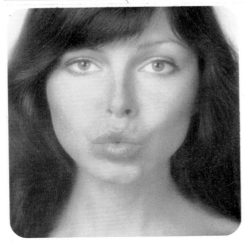 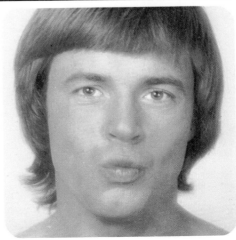

4

Helps to firm the jaw line

Shape your lips into an exaggerated rosebud-pout.
Do this 20 times.

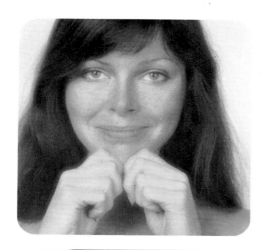

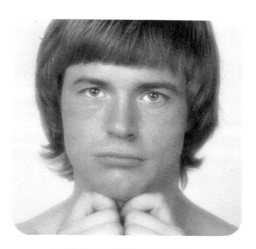

5

Stimulates the circulation around the jaw line and helps to prevent a double chin

Make a fist of each hand and, starting from the chin, pinch the flesh along the jaw line between the thumb and forefinger.

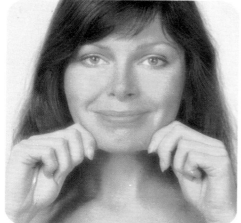

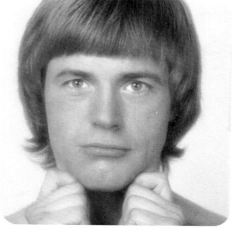

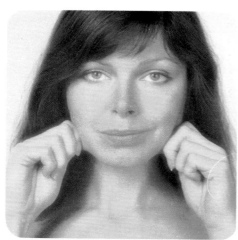

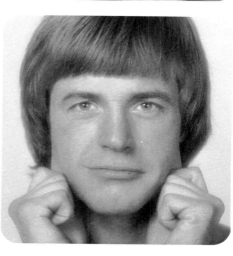

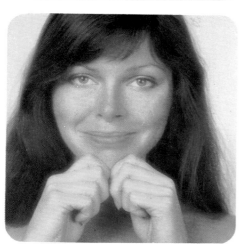

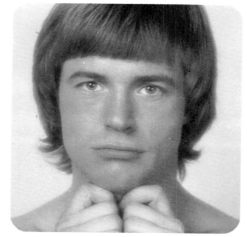

When you reach the end of the jawbone, work backwards once more from your chin.

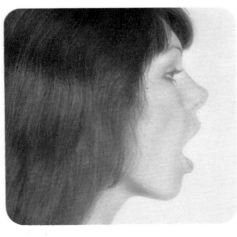
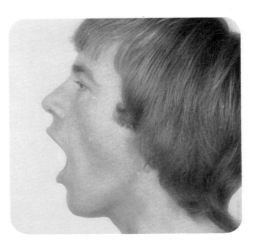

6
Firms the jaw, chin and throat

Open your mouth as wide as you can.

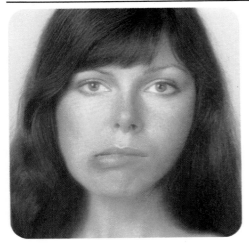
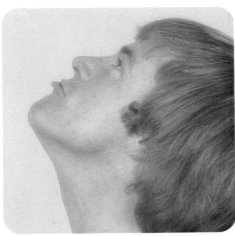

Let your head fall backwards, then stretch your lower lip over the upper lip as if you are trying to make it touch your nose. Hold for a mental count of five, feeling the tautness of the throat muscles.
Do this five times.

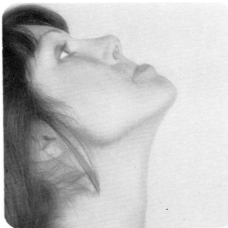
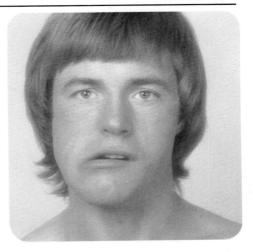

7
Strengthens jaw muscles and relaxes jaw

Push your lower jaw forward without straining and, keeping your head level, move your lower jaw to the right.

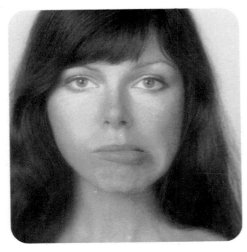
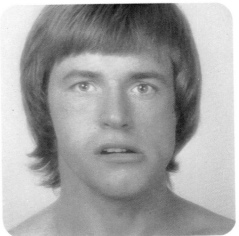

Move your jaw to the left as smoothly as possible.
Repeat this, moving the jaw rhythmically from side to side, 10 times to each side.

Keep Your Face Fit-2

The skin around your eyes, like the rest of your face, can be helped by exercise.

These exercises help to reduce the puffiness which may result from too little sleep. They stimulate the circulation around the eyes, including the corners where wrinkles first appear. The skin around the eyes is very delicate and tends to become dry, and improved circulation makes it more supple. These exercises also help to release tension and soothe your eyes.

Blinking is the natural way in which the eyes refresh themselves because it helps to bathe the eyes with tear fluid. You blink instinctively at regular intervals, whether you realize it or not. But if your eyes feel dry, prickly and tired, from reading too much or watching television, it can be very soothing to make a conscious effort to blink rapidly for a few seconds.

When your eyes are tired, close them and hold against them pads of cotton wool which have been soaked in hand-hot water and squeezed out. After a few seconds remove the pads and splash the area around the eyes with cool water. Repeat this three times.

Women should remove their eye make-up before doing these exercises. If your skin feels very taut when you do them, apply a little light cream around the eyes.

The Eyes

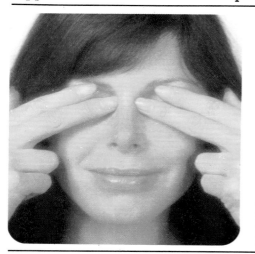

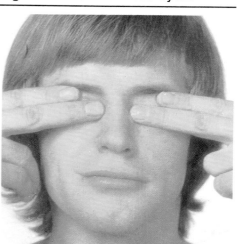

1

Strengthens the eyelids and counteracts crêpiness

Sit comfortably upright on a straight chair, elbows resting on a table. Close your eyes and place two fingers of each hand horizontally across each eyelid. Pretend you are trying to open your eyes against the very slight pressure of your fingers.
Do this three times.

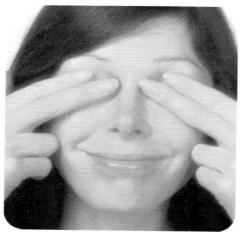

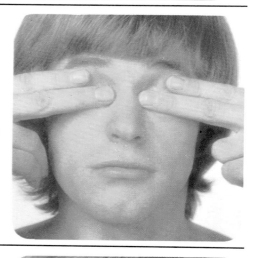

2

Strengthens eyelids and increases suppleness beneath the eyebrows

Sit upright, elbows on the table, with your eyes closed and two fingers horizontally over each eye. Raise your eyebrows against the slight pressure of your fingers.
Do this six times.

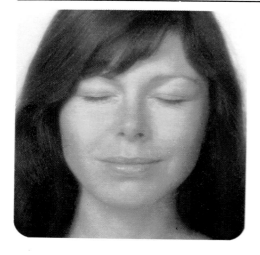

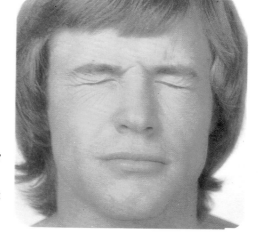

3

Strengthens upper and lower eyelids.

Slowly and with concentration blink hard.
Do this six times.

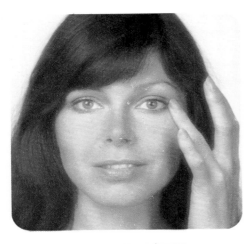

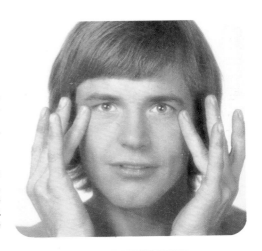

4

Stimulates circulation, reduces under-eye puffiness and counter-acts crow's-feet
Exercise both eyes at once or each in turn

Starting at the outer corners of the eyes and working towards the nose, "fingerprint" beneath your eyes with your ring finger which you have dipped in a little light face cream.

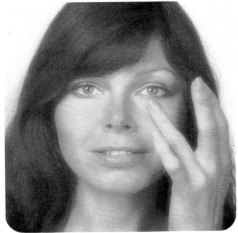

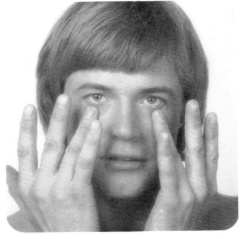

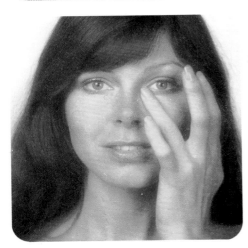

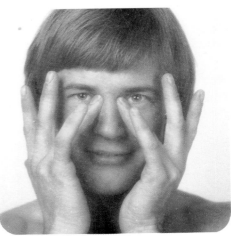

When you reach your nose, work outwards along the crease of the lids and back to where you began.

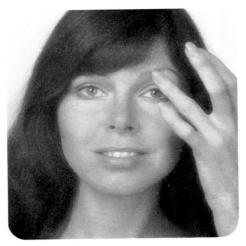

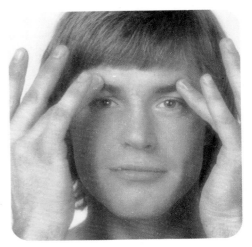

Do this exercise six times for each eye.

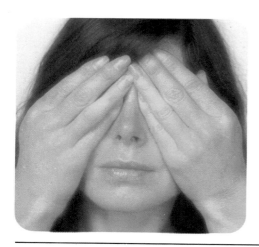

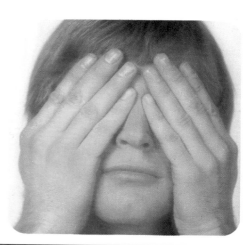

5

Helps to strengthen the eyelids, stimulates circulation and rests and brightens tired eyes

Sit upright, elbows on the table. Close your eyes and cup one hand over each eye.
Keep your eyes closed to a mental count of six and imagine that you are looking at black velvet.
Open your eyes and keep them open to a count of six. Then blink rapidly to a count of six, still keeping your eyes covered.
Do this exercise three times.

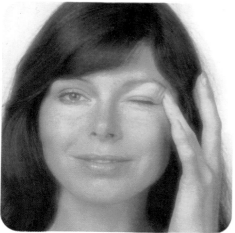

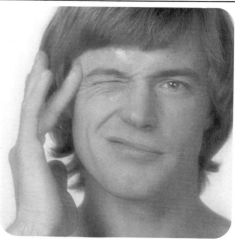

6

Strengthens the upper and lower lids

Find the muscle at the front of one temple by touching the temple with your ring finger and feeling where it contracts when you blink. Touch the temple with your finger gently, but firmly enough to feel the pressure. Wink the eye slowly but firmly.
Do this six times with each eye.

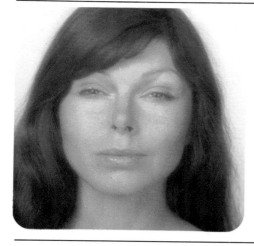

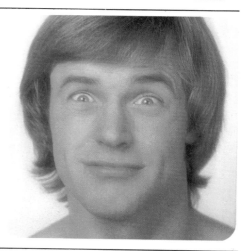

7

Helps to strengthen the lower eyelids and reduce puffiness

Raise your eyebrows and concentrate as hard as you can on raising the lower lids. Slightly lower the eyebrows and upper lids so that you are looking through narrowed eyes.
Do this six times.

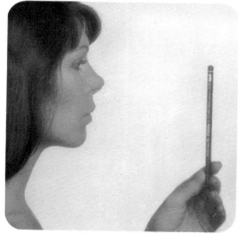

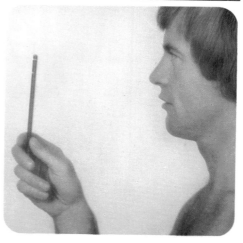

8

Reduces puffiness, strengthens eye muscles

Hold a pencil at eye level and about 10 inches from your eyes. Focus your eyes on the end of the pencil. Now change your focus to concentrate on a point on the wall beyond the pencil so that you are conscious of seeing two images of the pencil. Change your focus back to the pencil.
Do the exercise four times.

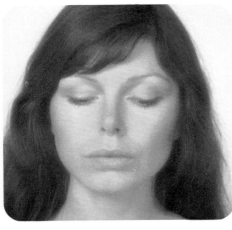

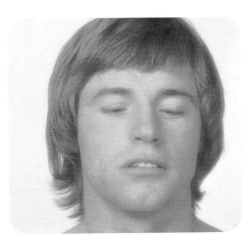

9
Relaxes the eyes and reduces puffiness

Keeping your head absolutely straight and still, concentrate on looking as far down as you can.

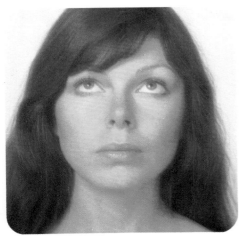

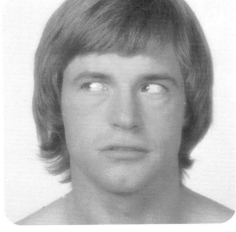

Look to the right as far as you can.

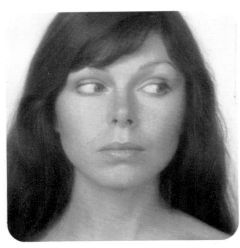

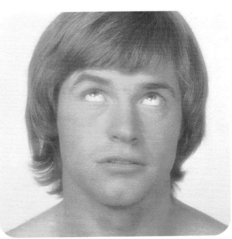

Look up as far as you can.

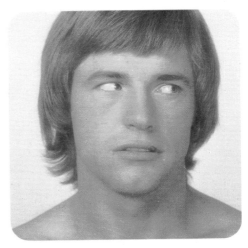

Look to the left as far as you can. Do the whole exercise five times.

Keep Your Face Fit-3

Your head weighs about 10 to 12 pounds. It is held in position by the strong muscles at the back of the neck, rather than by the weaker muscles at the front. If you habitually let your head poke forward or sag towards your chest, the muscles at the back of the neck will eventually weaken. You should always make an effort to keep your head balanced and upright, so that it is held in place by the muscles which are meant for the job.

These exercises, which tone up the muscles of the neck and shoulders, also help to improve posture. And because they help to relax tense muscles in the neck and shoulders, the exercises can also be useful in relieving headaches which are caused by fatigue and tension.

Neck and Shoulders

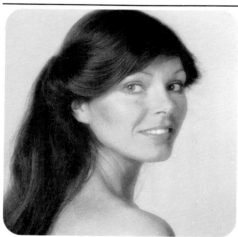

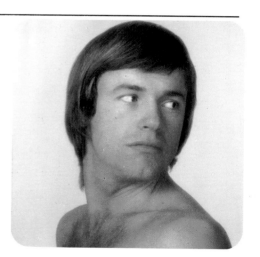

1

Increases suppleness of shoulders and improves posture

Sit relaxed but upright on a chair, facing forwards. Slowly turn your head as far as possible to one side, until you are looking backwards over your shoulder.

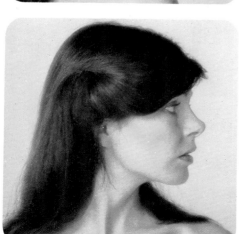

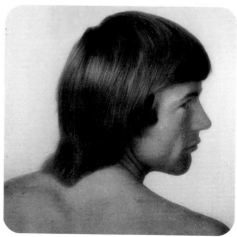

Relax, then repeat the exercise, turning to the other side.
Do the exercise three times to each side.

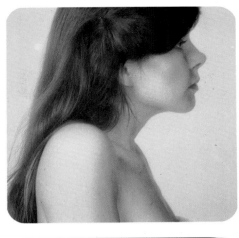

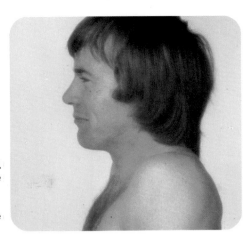

2

Helps poise, relieves tension and increases circulation in the shoulder area

Stand up straight and relax. Raise your shoulders towards your ears.

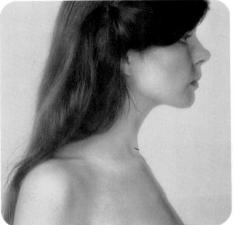

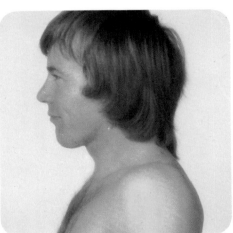

Rolling your shoulders as smoothly as you can, move them backwards.

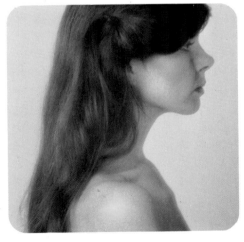

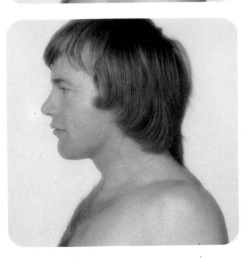

Then roll your shoulders downwards.

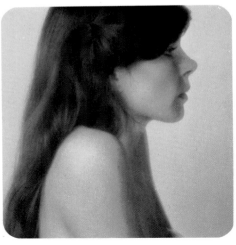

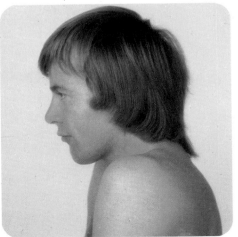

Roll your shoulders forwards and then up again.
Do the whole exercise smoothly and rhythmically five times. Relax.

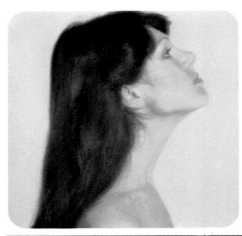

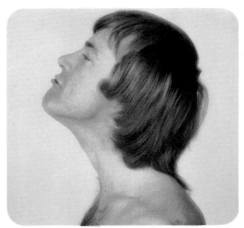

3

Strengthens the throat muscles

Sit relaxed but upright on a chair, facing forwards. Tilt your head back slightly, then push your jaw forwards and tense the neck muscles hard. Then lift your jaw higher and concentrate on feeling that you are trying to lift your neck out of your shoulders.
Do this five times.

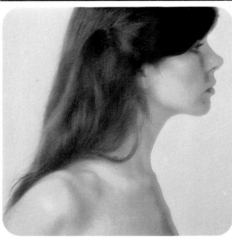

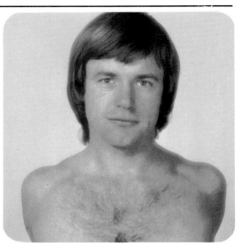

4

Strengthens shoulder muscles and makes them supple

Sit upright on a chair with your head straight and your arms relaxed. Join your hands loosely behind your back. Pull your shoulder-blades back hard, as though you are trying to make them meet. Feel the muscles contract.
Do this three times, relaxing only slightly in between. Then relax fully.

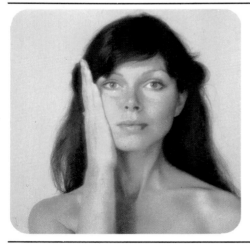

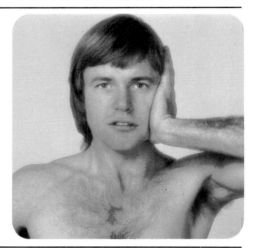

5

Strengthens the neck muscles

Place the flat of your hand along the side of your face. Hold this position firmly for a moment, then, using the muscles of your head, neck and shoulder, press as hard as you can with your head against your hand.
Do this five times on each side.

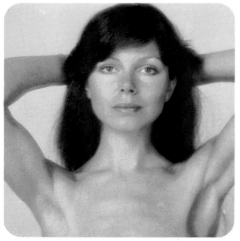

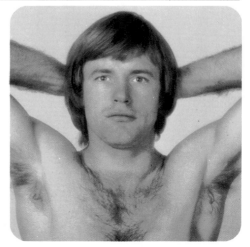

6

Strengthens the muscles at the side and the back of the neck

Clasp your hands behind your head. Press back against your hands as hard as you can.
Do this five times.

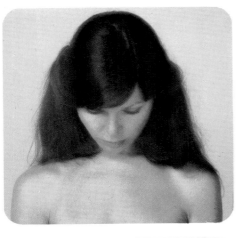

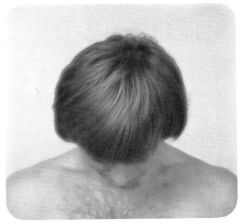

7
Releases tension, stimulates circulation and strengthens the neck muscles

Lower your chin on to your chest.

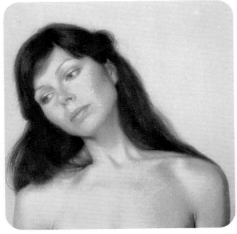

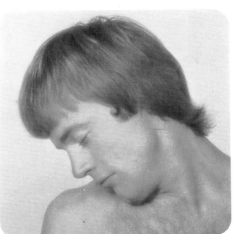

Roll your head to the right.

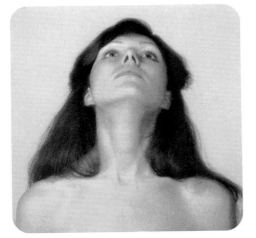

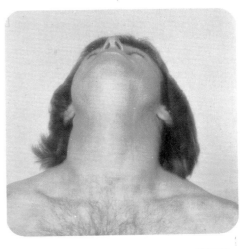

Roll your head backward.

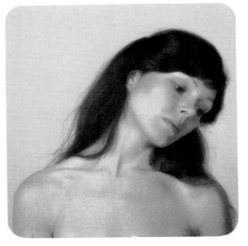

Roll your head to the left, and finish back in the starting position, with your head on your chest.
The whole exercise should be one slow, smooth movement. It should be done rhythmically three times in each direction.

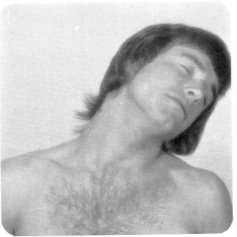

Care for Your Feet

Neglect your feet and it shows—on your face. Sadly, one of the most useful parts of the human anatomy is also one of the least well cared-for. Most people wait until foot troubles become unbearable before tackling the problem. But a little thought and careful choice of shoes can ensure that you do not suffer any of the unpleasant symptoms of foot neglect.

It is a pity that feet are so unloved, because beautiful, shapely ankles and perfectly formed toes can be as attractive as pretty hands. Feet are covered for most of the year, so the appeal of smooth, pampered feet is often forgotten. In summer, however, it is a different story for feet are on show. Open sandals or the bare-foot look on the beach can reveal a lifetime of neglect. Fortunately, although it is wisest to begin foot care in childhood, it is never too late to start looking after your feet.

Children's feet
The kicking enjoyed by tiny babies is their first foot and ankle exercises—and it helps to make feet and legs strong. (Mothers should never tuck bedclothes in so tightly that their baby cannot kick and bootees should be loose enough to allow toes to wriggle freely.) At birth, a child's feet consist of soft, small bones which do not become hardened fully until he or she is about 18 years old.

Tight nylon socks, badly-fitting shoes and slippers—even tight ballet pumps—all can help to deform the soft bones. Many children have wide feet and broad toes, so it is essential to measure width as well as length when fitting new shoes. A child should never wear rubber boots all day as these are very bad for the feet. They do not support the arch of the foot and could lead to flat feet later on. Another taboo is the slip-on type of shoe which has no support across the top or around the ankle. The natural action of the child is to curl his toes under to hold on the shoe, and this can result in permanently bent toes. To give feet maximum freedom for correct growth, small children should be allowed to go barefoot as much as possible in the house, on the beach or in the garden.

Teenagers' feet
As feet grow, they change their shape and proportion. It is, therefore, vital to continue checking foot measurements well into the teens before buying shoes. Fashion can be a big help—or hindrance—to healthy foot development in this age-group. Very narrow, pointed shoes and shoes with very high heels are extremely bad for teenage feet since the toes are squashed down into the front of the shoe and deformed in the process. Flatter shoes with a wide toe section are better, provided there is sufficient support on the instep.

One of the chief dangers for growing teenagers is foot infection. Verrucae are sometimes picked up in swimming pools or communal showers, and athlete's foot, which is caused by a fungus growth attacking the feet, can be contracted in places where warm, moist conditions lower skin resistance. Infections like these need professional treatment by a doctor or chiropodist, as they can be painful and also tend to spread if not caught at an early stage.

Adults' feet
It is hard to imagine yourself unable to go out to the shops because your feet are too painful to take you there, but this does happen to very many old people. And the main cause is usually neglect in the middle years of life. Bad shoes, tight socks or stockings and lack of general cleanliness and care can cause all kinds of problems.

Basic foot care involves keeping feet scrupulously clean, cutting toe-nails regularly and lavishing a little of the attention you normally pay to your hands to your feet as well.

If chilblains are your problem, massage your feet gently with a foot oil or lanolin. In hot weather use a special foot deodorant spray and put talcum powder in your shoes to prevent odour. Rinse stockings or tights nightly or wear clean socks every day. Never roast your feet over the fire in winter or sleep with your feet on a hot water bottle; these are the most common causes of chilblains.

After an exceptionally tiring day, 'paddle' your feet in cold, salted water. This is better than the traditional mustard bath which softens the skin too much. After bathing, always dry your feet carefully between the toes. And choose your slippers carefully, do not wear casual 'mules' all day, they don't give enough arch support.

For every day, choose shoes that allow your toes to move freely, and that grip the heel and instep firmly. When buying shoes, walk up and down in the shop several times before deciding if they fit properly and are comfortable. Shoes should not have to be worn in, they should fit straight away. Beware of wooden-soled shoes as these can be harmful to the arch of the foot.

Don't be brave about minor foot ailments, be sensible instead. Chiropodists spend much of their time sorting out problems caused by their patients' attempts at self-medication, the damage done can be very grave indeed. Never poke at corns or hard skin with a razor, nail file or other unsterilized instrument. Don't use corn solvents yourself or

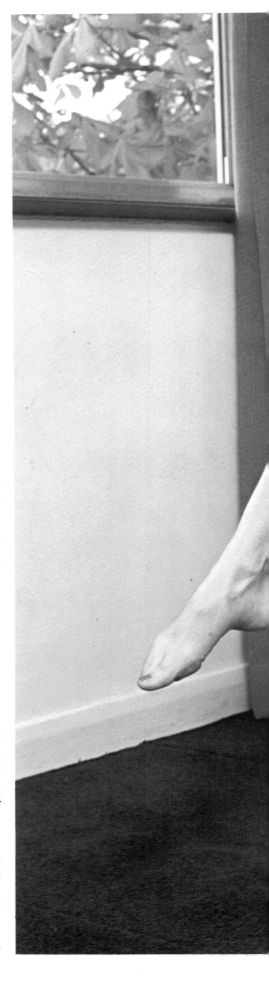

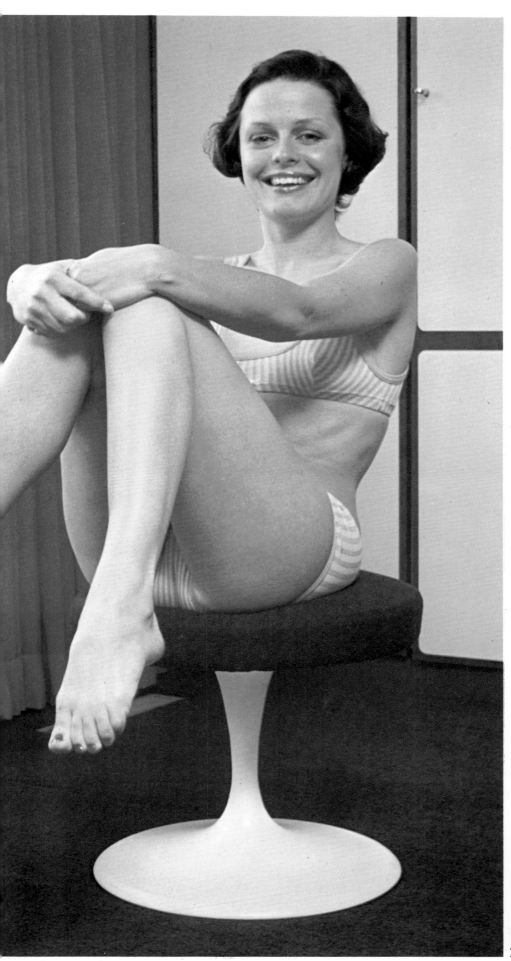

attempt to apply a lambs' wool protection for the toe as this can easily restrict circulation. A 15-minute foot check-up twice a year is an excellent idea. And if corns, callouses or more serious foot ailments develop, then professional treatment is essential.

Chiropody has a 'middle-aged' image —but young people too can benefit tremendously from the services of a good chiropodist. Don't think that a single, nagging corn is too unimportant for you to take professional advice about. It is better to deal with minor problems as they occur than to suffer for 20 years and then present a chiropodist with a full range of foot ailments.

Exercises For The Feet

EXERCISE 1
Strengthens ankles.

Sit on a stool or the edge of the bed. Raise your legs and bend your knees, clasping your hands round your knees for support. Now rotate your feet first outwards and then inwards. Repeat for a few minutes.

EXERCISE 2
Strengthens ankles.

In the same position as 1 point your toes alternately upwards and downwards. Repeat 30 times.

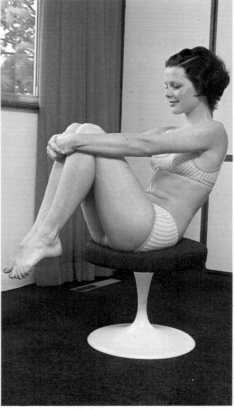

1

2

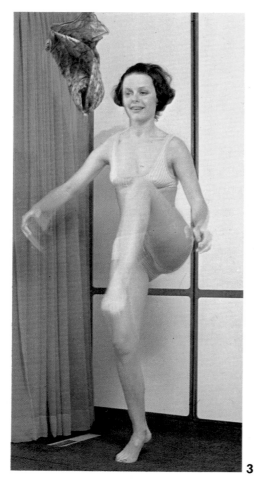

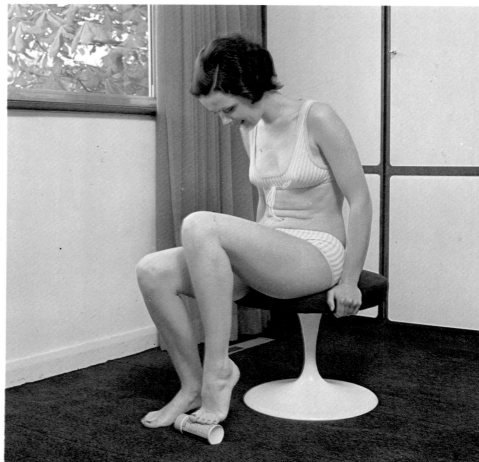

3

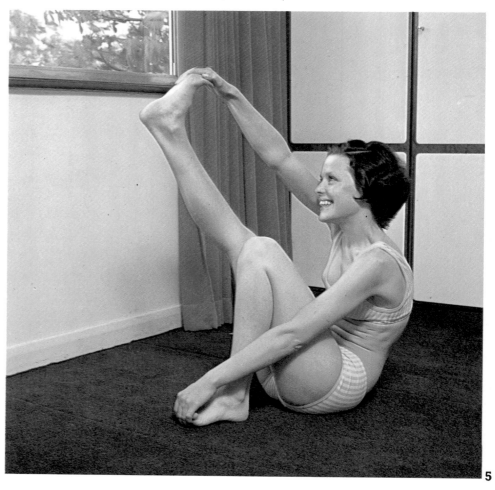

4

5

EXERCISE 3
Strengthens toes and arches.

In a standing position throw a light
scarf or handkerchief in the air and
keep it there by kicking with
alternate feet. Repeat 10 times or
until tired.

EXERCISE 4
**Strengthens arches and balls
of feet.**

Sit on a stool or the edge of the bed.
Place a cylinder such as an aerosol
can of hair-spray on the floor. Put
your right foot on the can and roll it
backwards and forwards from the
tips of the toes to the heel. Now use
the left foot. Repeat five times with
each foot.

EXERCISE 5
Strengthens toes and ankles.

Sit on the floor, with your knees
bent and your back straight. Clasp
your right foot with your right hand
and your left foot with your left
hand. Now raise left and right feet
alternately in a scissors movement.
Repeat 10 times.

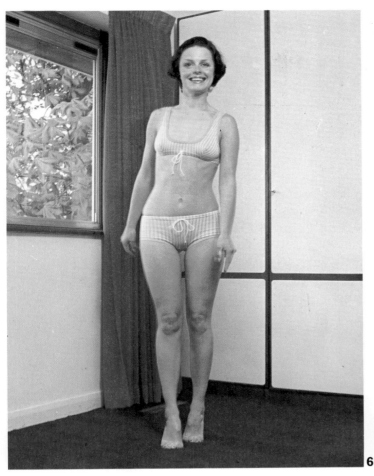

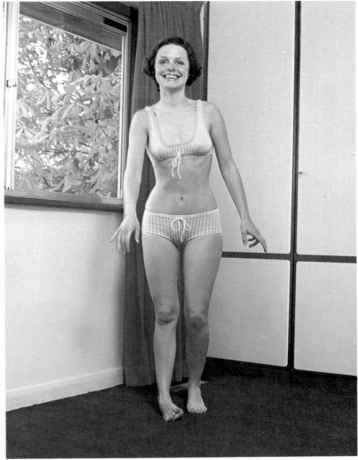

EXERCISE 6
Increases circulation and strengthens feet and ankles.

Stand at one end of the room. Take four paces on tip-toe, four on your heels, four on the inside of your feet, four on the outside. Relax and walk backwards in the same way.

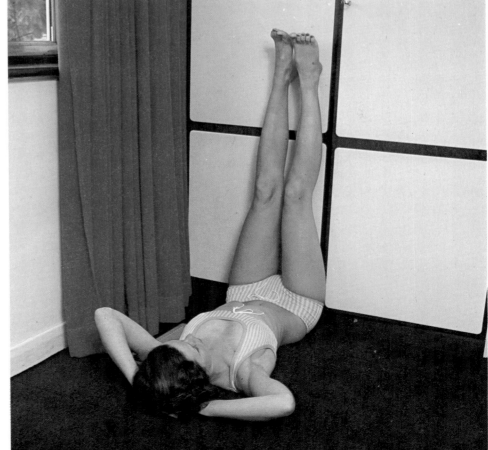

EXERCISE 7
Relaxes feet and legs when tired.

Lie on your back with your legs up against the wall. Try to form a right-angle with your legs and your body. Stay in this position until you feel refreshed.

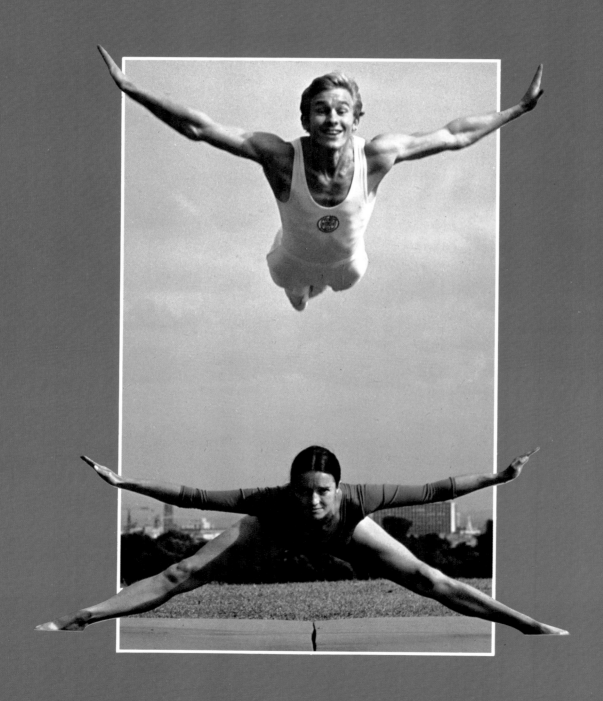

Gymnastics–1

Gymnastics is a precise sport and exercise routine. There is something really impressive about a person who can do cartwheels, tumbles, full turns, backward and forward rolls with consummate ease. So many people desire to imitate gymnasts and be as proficient as they are.

This four-part course teaches you the basic gymnastic movements in a simple, easy-to-follow way. You can learn them in the comfort of your own home, in a local park or in your garden if the weather permits.

Many gymnastic movements look more difficult than they really are. This is because a movement—such as a cartwheel—is always seen as a whole. But each movement can be broken down into a number of recognizable component parts. Once you know these different parts and can see the way one automatically follows another the whole movement becomes much easier and more accessible.

This course breaks down each movement into precise and exact detail. By following the instructions and pictures carefully you will be surprised at the ease with which you learn gymnastics. And you can learn step by step, at your own speed.

What benefits can gymnastics give you? First of all, a gymnastic routine is a showpiece by which you can entertain friends and it is also an excellent form of exhilarating recreation. And gymnastics is now recognized as a systematized form of physical exercise, not only fascinating to watch but also of high therapeutic value. It offers a means of developing the discipline of your body and mind. It will teach you to co-ordinate the working of all your muscles in a graceful and balanced way. Your whole body is toned up and you will feel so much healthier. Gymnastics also shows you how to focus your power of concentration so that you will learn to think and react more quickly, gaining a valuable system of mental discipline.

These and other benefits account for the present popularity of gymnastics. The high skills displayed by the competitors in recent Olympic Games and other international competitions have demonstrated the natural agility and poise of those who practise gymnastics, causing an upsurge of interest in the sport among people who realize that they can also learn the grace and balance of the gymnast.

What clothing is most suitable for practising the gymnastic movements? The prime consideration is that no matter what you wear it should be light and cause no hindrance to your movements. A bikini or a pair of shorts and a T-shirt are suitable. The best clothing is a leotard for women and a jumpsuit for men (shown by the models in the pictures). Both of these pieces of clothing are cheap and can be bought in any sports shop. It is also advisable to wear some kind of shoes—at least while you are learning.

The course starts with the basic forward roll, backward roll and side roll. Also included are the straddle stand, the one leg stand, the half turn and a springing exercise. The later parts of the course will teach you how to make these basic movements more colourful to do and fascinating to watch. When you have progressed through all the movements the course will show you how to put some of the movements together into an attractive, flowing routine.

Practise each part of the course as much as you can. The more time you devote to learning the sooner you will become proficient. The most important thing is to remember to follow the progression of the movements. Never move on to another movement until you have perfected the previous one. And pay close attention to each part of a movement. Perfecting each separate part will make the whole movement look more masterly.

Posture and balance are important for the movements. The correct posture is achieved by distributing the weight of your body evenly between the feet. You should lean neither forwards nor backwards. When you master this kind of posture your sense of balance will automatically improve.

Do not worry if you find balance slightly difficult at first. You will become better as your fitness improves and you are more relaxed. If you have special trouble with balance, practise the one leg stand more than any of the other movements. You will soon master it.

Never relax your muscles while you are going through a movement. Otherwise it will not be as efficient and spritely as you would want it to be. This applies to the starting position as much as it does to the other movements. Always keep your body taut, your muscles tight and your mind alert so that you are ready to spring into action with style and grace.

Make a resolution to start this four-part course at the easiest time you can arrange. Early in the morning or late at night are usually the most convenient. The course gives you a guarantee of continued fitness, if you follow it for any length of time.

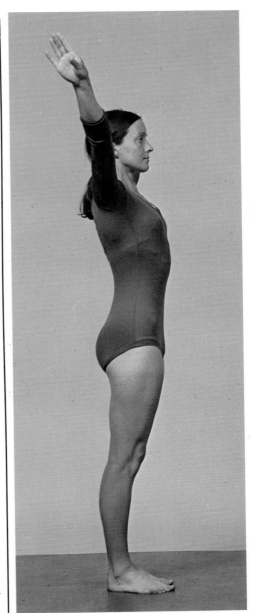

STARTING POSITION
Gymnastics requires a great degree of poise and balance. And this can only be achieved by a correct starting position and concentration while you are going through one of the movements. The starting position for all of the movements in this course is the same and should be used every time you attempt a movement. Each movement should also finish with the same position.
Stand with your feet together. Keep your legs close to each other. Make sure your muscles are tight. Pull the stomach in and hold your shoulders well back and relaxed. The head should be held level. Your arms can be either rested by your sides or stretched above the shoulders.
Hold this position for a few seconds to help you concentrate on the movement you are about to execute.

117

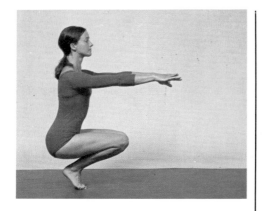

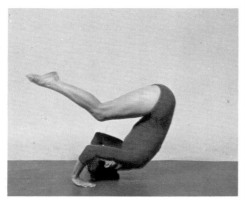

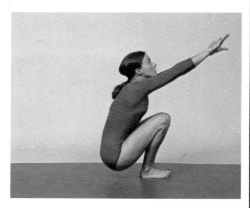

SIMPLE FORWARD ROLL

1. From standing in the starting position, crouch down on your toes. Keep your legs together and your thighs straight. Do not lean back on to your ankles. Place your hands on the floor, shoulder-width apart. Tuck your head into the chest and round your back. Push off the floor with your feet.

2. Taking your weight on your hands and, keeping the back rounded, bring your legs over your head and roll forward on your rounded back.

3. When your feet reach the floor, stretch your hands upwards over your head and lift your body off the floor to regain the position shown in picture one.

Finish in a standing position, legs and feet together and your arms outstretched.

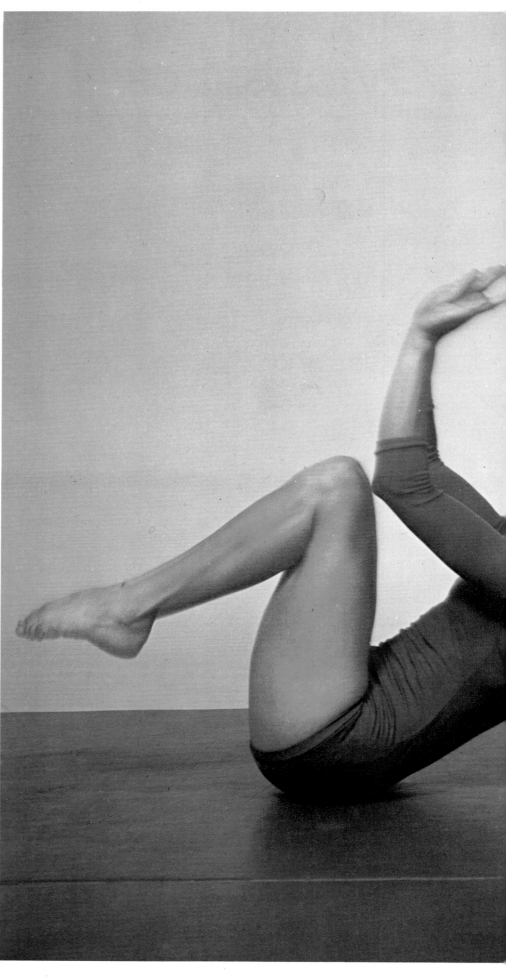

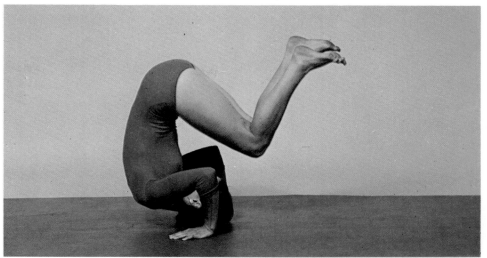

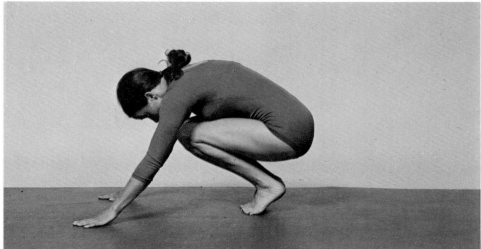

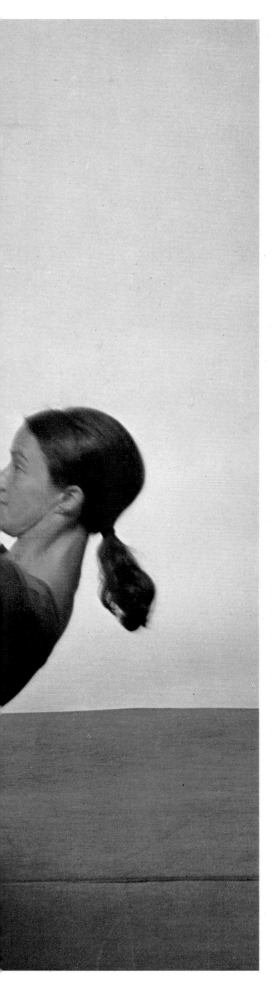

SIMPLE BACKWARD ROLL

1. From the starting position, bend your knees and balance on your toes. Stretch your arms in front of you. Do not lean back on your ankles. Hold your head straight. Roll backwards by first rounding your back, placing your chin close to the chest and then sitting on the floor. The roll continues backwards with the arms being carried over the head as your feet leave the floor.

2. Place your hands close to the shoulders and push to lift the hips over the head. Your head must pass between your hands. This can only be done by taking the weight of your body on your arms and pushing the arms as straight as possible. Keep your legs close to the body all the time.

3. Pushing on the arms, bring your feet on to the floor keeping the body curled. Place the toes on the floor.

4. Gently push your hands upwards and outwards away from the floor to bring the body upright and balanced on the toes. Keep your legs and feet together.

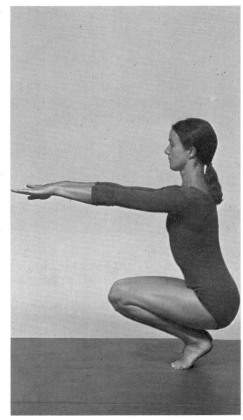

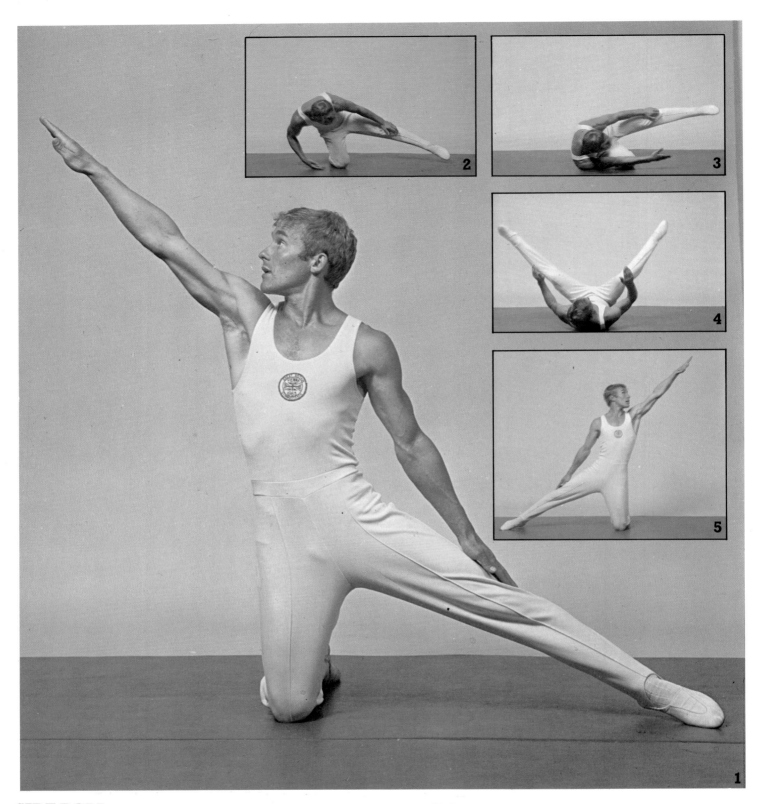

SIDE ROLL

1. Kneel on your right knee with your thigh and hip in a straight line with your shoulder. Stretch your left leg sideways to the left. Raise your right arm upwards obliquely and move your left arm downwards with your fingers resting on your left leg.

2. Fold your right arm under your shoulder and bend the body over slightly.

3. Roll sideways along the right arm, starting to move the left leg over. The left arm should follow the line of the left leg.

4. Continue the roll across the shoulders and back, keeping your left leg straight. Begin to lift the right leg off the floor.

As the roll progresses to the left, straighten your shoulders and bend the left leg inwards. Continue the roll on to the left arm, bringing the left leg into a kneeling position. The left arm should lift outwards and upwards while the right arm stretches downwards.

5. The right leg should be straightened. Shift the weight of your body on to your left knee. Stretch your left arm upwards obliquely and your right arm in line with your right leg. Hold this position for a few seconds before returning to the starting posture of standing straight.

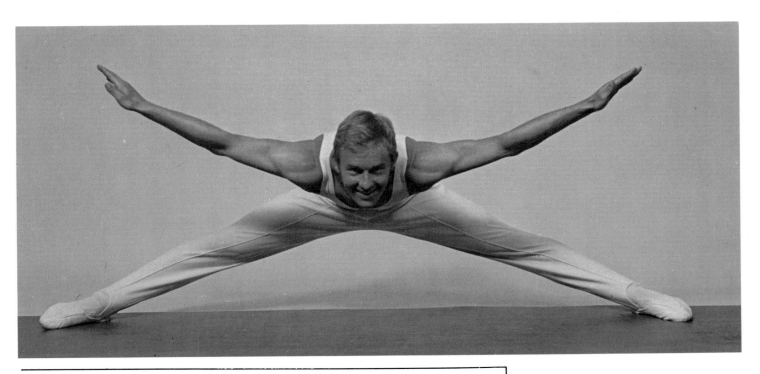

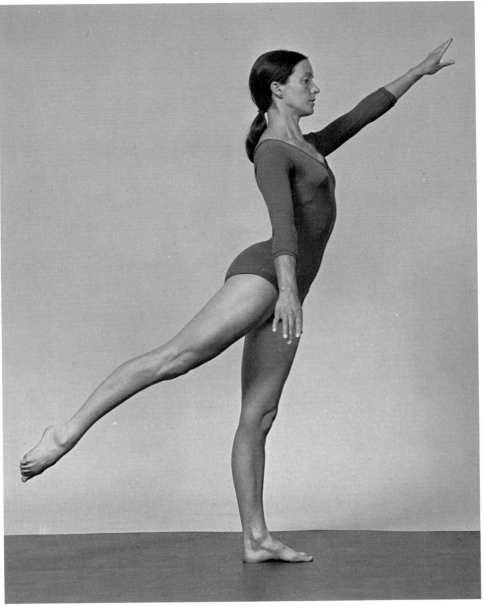

STRADDLE STAND
Place your feet wide apart with your legs and back straight. Point your toes outwards so that you are almost standing along the inside edges of your feet.
Keeping your legs, hips, shoulders and head in a straight line, stretch your arms upwards at 45° angles to your shoulders. The arms and legs should form a cross, with the left arm in line with the right leg and the right arm in line with the left leg. Now bend the body forwards as shown in the picture. Keep your back as straight as possible. Bend from the tops of the legs only. Stretch your arms sideways and upwards so that they are above the level of the back and held well back.

ONE LEG STAND
Stand on both legs and keep your body upright. Tighten the muscles of your legs and buttocks. Slide one leg backwards a few inches behind the other and point your toes. Keep your hips slightly forward all the time.
Slowly lift your leg off the floor. Do not swing or jerk as this will immediately put you off balance. Do not lift or twist the hips in order to raise your leg higher. Keep your spine as straight as possible and do not lean the top of the body forwards.
Keep the body stretching upwards and the shoulders down. Hold this position steady.

HALF TURN

The aim of this movement is to spring as high as possible without breaking the symmetry of your body.

1. From standing in the starting position, bend your knees and spring straight upwards.

Do not begin to turn your body until the feet have left the floor. Point your toes and keep the body upright.

2. Turn your head to look at where you intend to land. Keep your body turning with your head.

3. Land with your feet together, bending the knees slightly to absorb the landing. Finish by immediately stretching upwards. This movement is a preparation for the full turn. If you feel you can do the half turn with ease why not try a full turn? It becomes easier with each practice session.

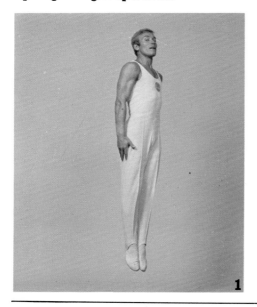

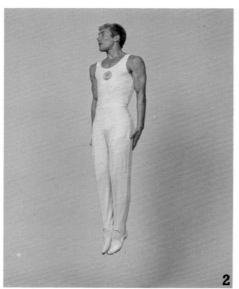

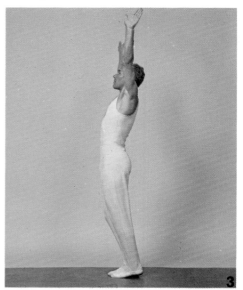

PLIĒS WITH SPRING

1. Stand with heels and legs together. Women should turn their toes out and keep their knees apart. Bend the knees, keeping the heels of your feet on the floor. The body should be kept upright.

2. Spring upwards without leaning backwards or forwards. Stretch your legs straight and point your toes.

Land with your feet flat on the floor, ready to start again. Repeat as many times as you wish.

It is important in this movement to keep the body straight when you spring upwards. Use your legs only to gain spring and height. Always wait to gain composure before repeating the movement.

This completes the first part of the Gymnastics course. You will find as you progress that these basic exercises cannot be practised enough as they will be constantly repeated in the combination exercises that follow. Therefore you will be well advised to practise until you feel completely at ease with these first steps and can perform them without any sign of strain. They should be completely automatic before you attempt any of the combinations in the latter part of the course. You will have already discovered the benefits of gymnastics to your health and general fitness, now enjoy the pleasure that well co-ordinated movement can bring, as you gain skill, poise and balance.

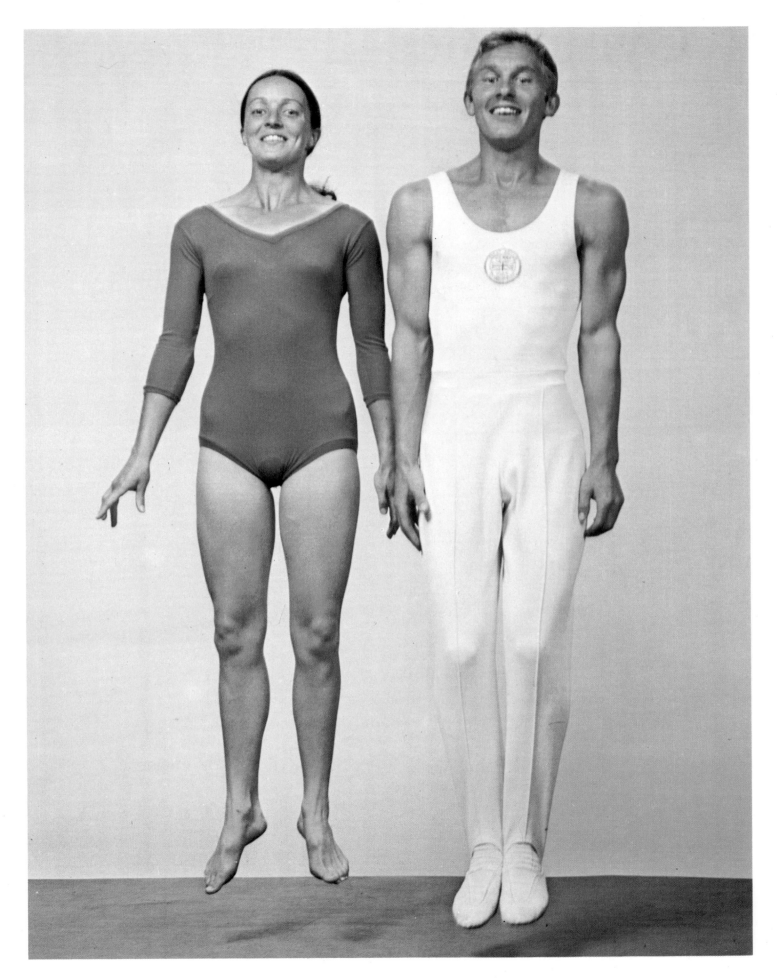

Gymnastics—2

The second part of the gymnastics course continues with a series of energetic jumps, a graceful arabesque, a simple headstand and some variations on the movements which you learned in *Gymnastics—1*. The new movements enable you to develop even more balance and poise while at the same time making you fitter and more relaxed.

Gymnastics has many in-built benefits for your health. Your breathing will deepen so that your circulation is greatly improved. Your spine and muscles will gain such a new degree of suppleness that you walk and carry yourself with more ease and dignity.

Each of the following movements give you specific benefits. The headstand teaches you to move slowly and calmly and is good for the health of your hair.

The arabesque instils a sense of easeful balance which can be called upon even when you are not doing gymnastics. The roll movements give you speed and co-ordination. And the various jumps inculcate in you a feeling of lightness and invigoration.

Remember that each movement must start and end with the starting position shown in *Gymnastics—1*. This posture gives you time to collect your thoughts so that you can concentrate all that much more while you are actually going through a movement.

Practise the movements as much as you can so that you can learn with ease the exercises in the next two parts.

Daily gymnastic practice sessions will give you a freshness that carries over into everyday life.

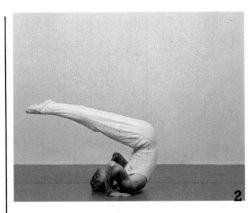

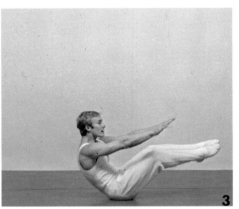

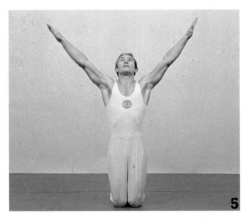

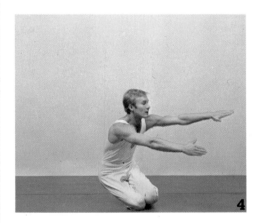

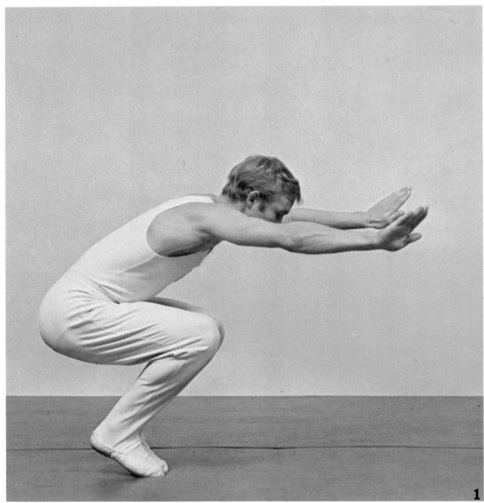

FORWARD ROLL TURN TO KNEEL

1. From the standing position, crouch down balancing on your toes. Reach forward with your arms and point your fingers outwards at a slight angle.

2. Place your hands on the floor and tuck your head close to your chest. Pushing with your hands, begin to roll along your back, keeping it rounded. Your legs should be straight as you roll.

3. As your buttocks reach the floor

bend your knees to one side. Reach your hands over your head.
4. Place your knees on the floor and push upwards, lifting the hips to your left.
5. Finish the movement by kneeling upright and stretching your arms.

BACKWARD ROLL TO STRADDLE STAND

1. Take up the starting position. Then bend forward from the hips, keeping your back as straight as you can. Move your hands towards the floor and reach backwards so that your arms pass your legs.

2. Keeping your legs straight, drop backwards and reach for the floor with your hands. Taking the weight of your body on your arms, let your buttocks and legs sink gently on to the floor. Your toes should be pointed.

3. Roll along your rounded back. At the same time, bring your hands over your head to place the palms close to the shoulders—fingers facing inwards. Keep your legs and hips lifting over.

4. Open your legs wide as your feet come close to the floor. Keep your legs straight.

5. Push strongly on your hands, lifting your head between your arms. Continue to raise your hips upwards. Push away from the floor with your hands and stretch the arms and body outwards and upwards. Finish the movement with your arms stretched obliquely up. Your legs, trunk and head should be held in a line. Hold this posture for a few seconds.

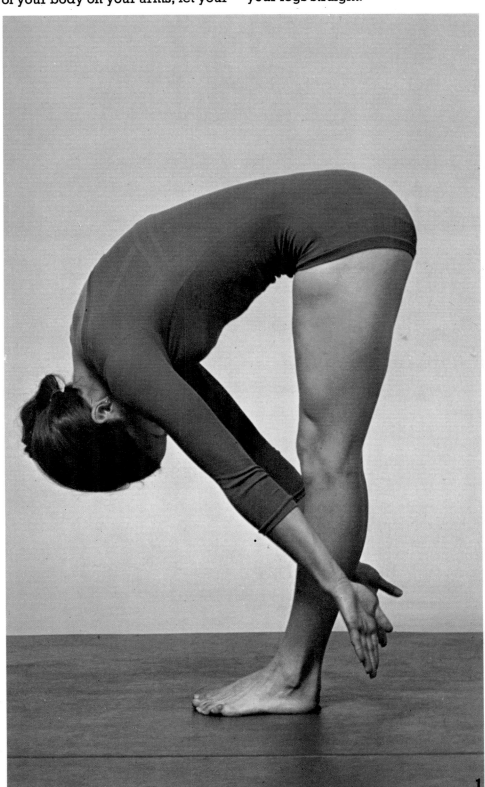

1

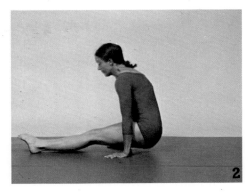

2

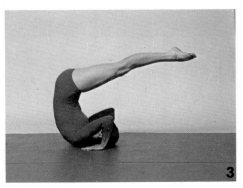

3

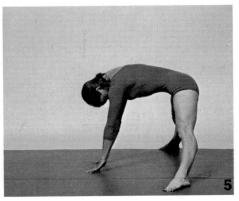

4

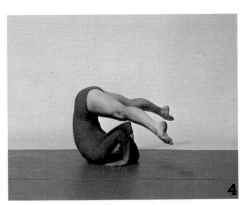

5

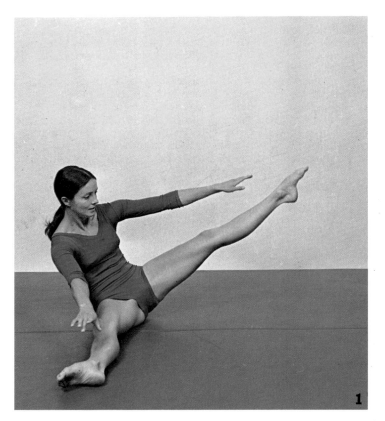

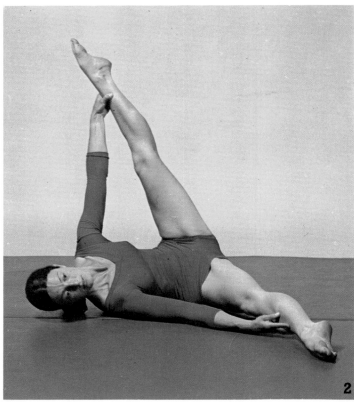

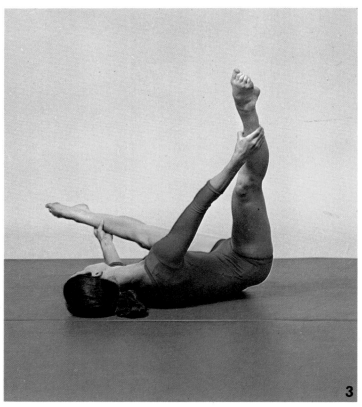

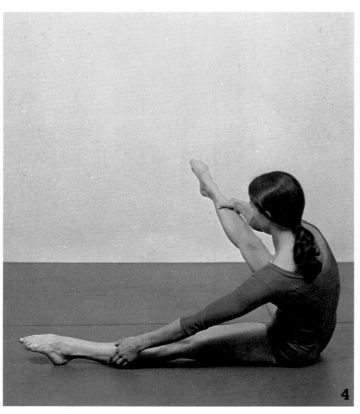

SIDE CIRCLE ROLL

1. Sit on the floor with your legs as far astride as possible. Press the back of your knees firmly against the floor. Point your toes. Holding your back as straight as you can, stretch your arms out towards your legs.

Decide whether you will find it easier to roll to the left or to the right. Lean to that side keeping the straddle sitting position. Lift the opposite leg off the floor.

2. Roll on to the shoulder and grasp your ankles as the legs lift. Keep your legs apart and straight.

3. Continue the roll across the back to the other shoulder with your legs following over the top.

4. Rise up to face in the opposite direction from which you started. The leading leg should reach the floor before the trailing leg. Finish the movement in the same position from which you started. Hold this position for a few seconds without relaxing your muscles or losing the tension of your body.

INVERTED BALANCE

1. From a standing start, kneel down with your toes tucked in. Place your hands on the floor, shoulder-width apart. Position the front of your head on the floor so that a triangle is formed with the hands. This makes a stable base to balance on.

Keeping the head still, straighten your legs sufficiently to bring the hips directly in line with the centre point between your hands and head. Hold the neck, shoulder and back muscles tight. All of your weight should be equally distributed between your hands and head.

2. Lift the toes from the floor. Do not jump. Bend the knees. Keep your legs pressed tightly together. Begin to straighten your legs as you move them upwards.

3. As your legs reach a straight position, transfer your weight distribution slightly by easing the hips forwards. The body weight should be perfectly balanced between the hands and the head. Hold this position for a few seconds. Finish the movement by coming down through the same stages and finally ending in your original kneeling position.

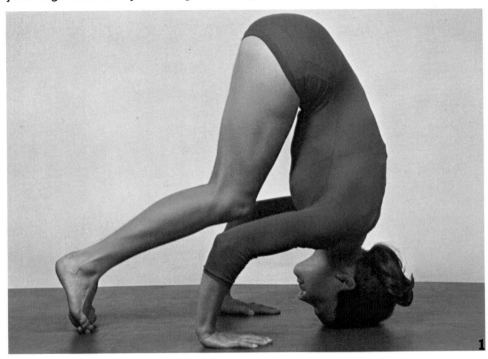

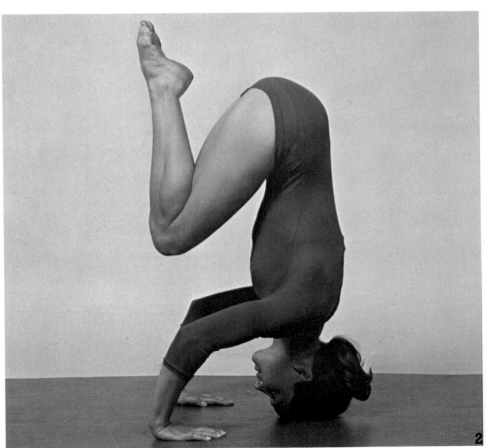

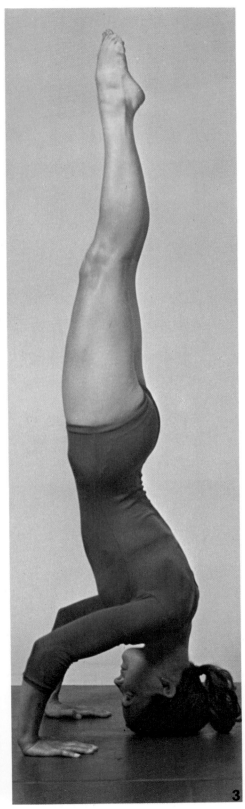

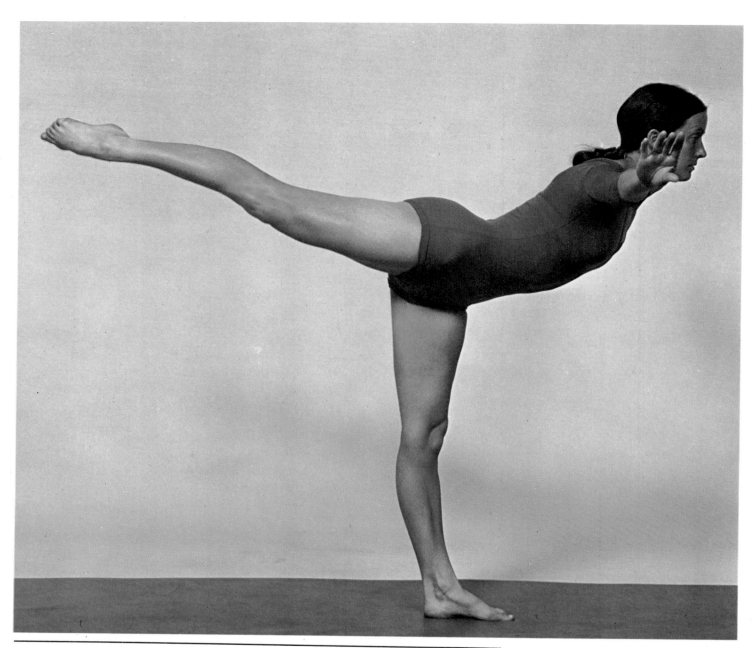

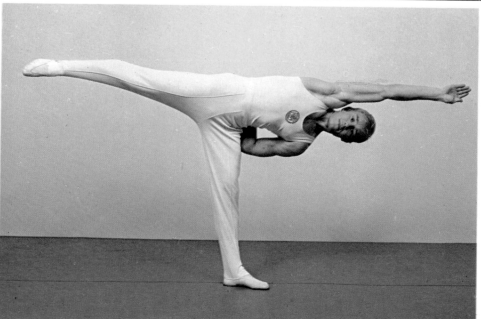

ARABESQUE
This posture is a progression from a one leg stand in *Gymnastics—1*. Go through the one leg balance once or twice more before trying this arabesque. It is important that you are able to maintain steady balance for a period of time. When you have taken up the one leg balance position, lift your right leg backwards and as high as you possibly can without unduly straining. Keep both legs straight.

SIDE BALANCE
A side balance must be executed very slowly. Do not start to lean over unless you have achieved a firm balance stance on one leg. When you are balanced on one leg, lean over to the left. Your top arm should reach over as you lift your leg. Tuck the lower arm behind your back. Do not lean forwards or backwards.

SCISSOR JUMP

Take one step then jump, swinging your arms as the jump commences to gain height. Your legs must be straight throughout and your toes pointed. Swing the legs upwards one before the other and switch direction in mid-air. Land on the leg which did not start the jump. Repeat a few times in succession.

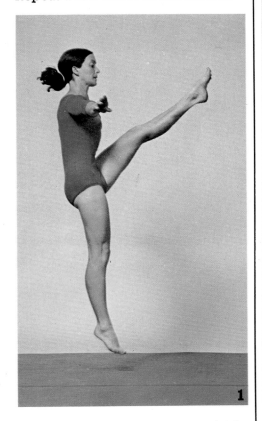

1

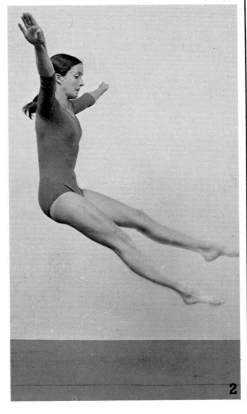

2

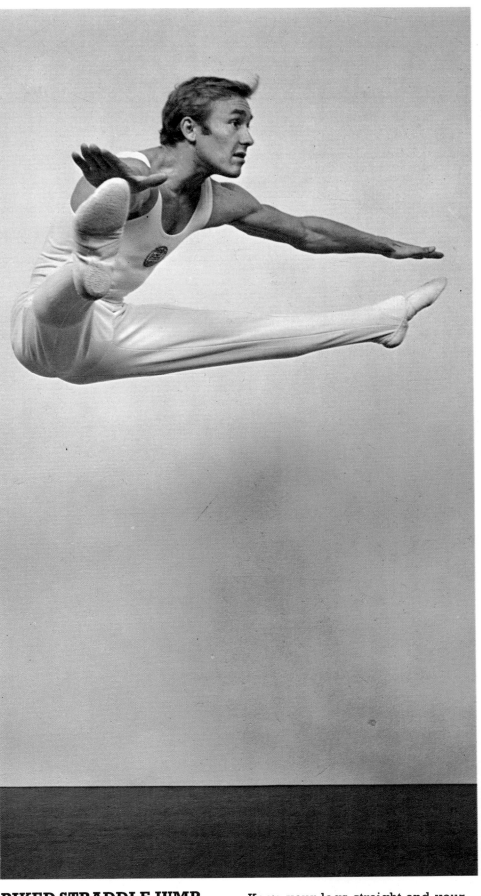

PIKED STRADDLE JUMP

Take two or three paces and leap upwards from a two-foot take-off. Straddle your legs and stretch your arms out towards your feet. Keep your legs straight and your back as erect as possible. Do not try to gain too much height when you start to learn this movement.

Gymnastics—3

This, the third part of the gymnastics course, contains the movements which are so exciting and stimulating to see performed by professional gymnasts. They often look difficult but with some practice you too can learn to do them. You will gain much more enjoyment from actually doing a cartwheel, a handstand, a crab or a roll than from just being a spectator.

Decide to practise the movements daily and you will be surprised at the speed with which you learn them. The pictures and the instructions are designed for simplicity and ease. Each movement is broken down into its basic parts so that you can go through it step by step knowing exactly what to do, how to do it and how to spot any mistakes you may make so that you can easily eliminate them.

It is a good idea to learn a movement each day. You can devote one practice session to learning the forward roll to straddle, another to the backward roll with straight legs, the third and fourth days to the handstand and the cartwheel, and so on. This is not absolutely necessary, but you may find it easier to learn them in this way.

Gymnastics is an entertaining sport as well as being a precise system of physical movement. So above all enjoy yourself when you are practising. Even your initial mistakes can be a source of enjoyment as well as being educational. Everyone can learn from their mistakes.

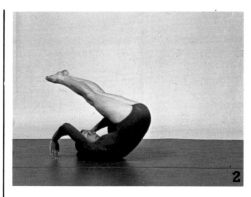

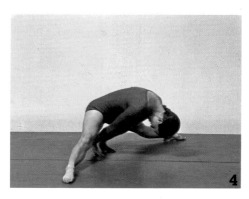

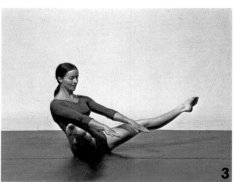

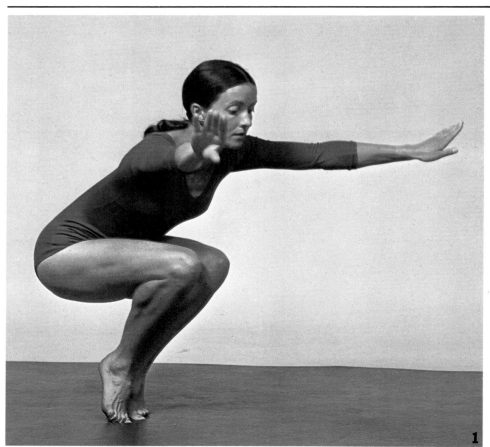

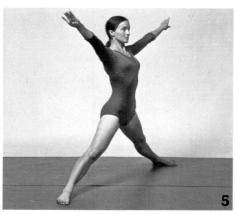

FORWARD ROLL TO STRADDLE

Each movement should begin and end with the starting position described in Gymnastics—1. This will help you compose your mind and focus your concentration on the movement which you are about to perform.

1. From the starting position, crouch down and balance on your toes.

2. Place your hands on the floor well in front of your body. At the same time push from your toes with your legs together. Tuck your head into your chest, roll onto your shoulders, keeping your legs straight as your feet leave the floor.

3. Roll along your back with your legs straight and close to your body. Straddle your legs and bring your hands to the floor between your legs as close as possible to your body. Keep your muscles tensed, ready for the next movement.

4. Keeping your head tucked in, press down on your hands and lean forwards until your hips are in line with your feet.

5. Lift your hands off the floor, reach forwards and straighten your back. Finish by bringing your body upright and stretching your arms to the side and above your shoulders.

BACKWARD ROLL WITH STRAIGHT LEG

The first movements of this exercise are similar to the first three parts of the backward roll to straddle stand shown in Gymnastics—2. Go through these again and then proceed as follows.

1. Keeping your legs straight and together bring them over your head. Place your feet on the floor close to your hands. Push your arms and lift your head.

2. Push your arms straight to bring your hips and legs into a vertical line.

Finish by lifting your arms from the floor and stretching upwards and outwards until your body is in a straight line with your arms which are raised above your head.

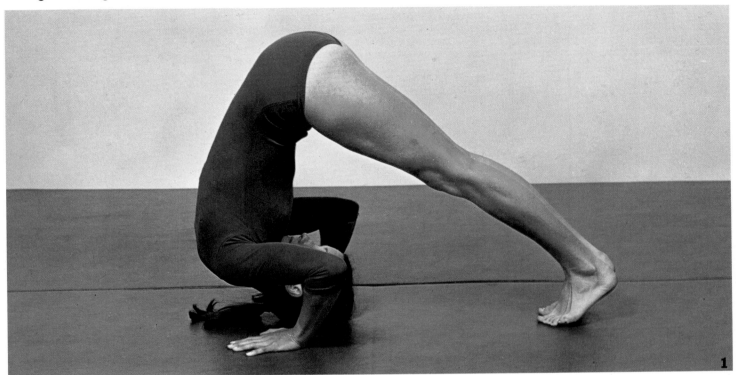

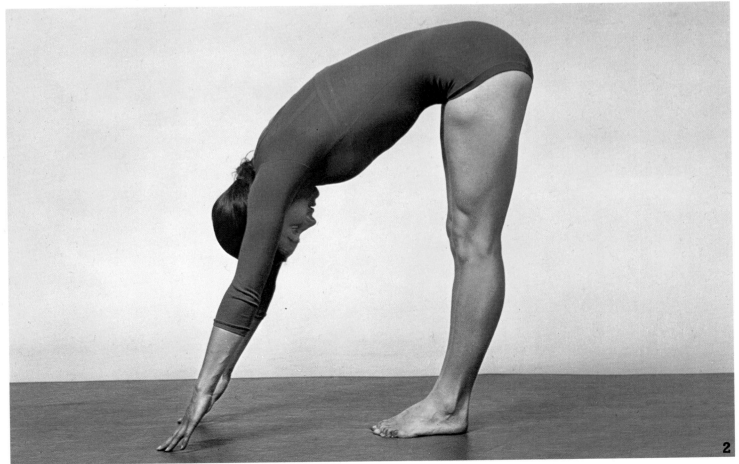

BACKWARD ROLL TO HANDSTAND

1. From a standing start, bend forwards sharply placing your arms behind your legs with your hands close to the floor and your fingers outstretched.
2. Drop backwards onto your hands keeping your body bent and your toes pointed.
3. Roll onto your back bringing your hands behind your shoulders and placing them flat on the floor with your fingers pointing backwards.

When your legs reach a point just past the vertical, drive your body upwards towards the ceiling. This is done by pushing up from your hips and at the same time thrusting upwards through your shoulders and arms.
4. Keep thrusting upwards until your arms are perfectly straight or 'locked out'. Your leg muscles must also be held in tension and the muscles in your buttocks should be squeezed tightly together in order to maintain balance. Your stomach and back muscles must also be working to help keep your balance. In the handstand position your hands, back, hips and legs are in a straight line and your toes are pointed. Hold this position for as long as you feel at ease.

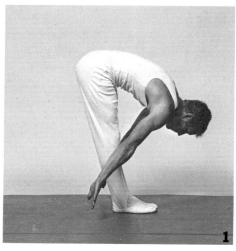

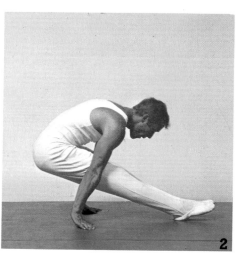

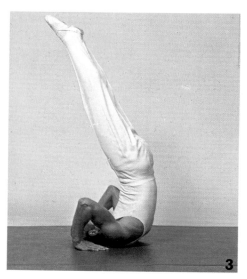

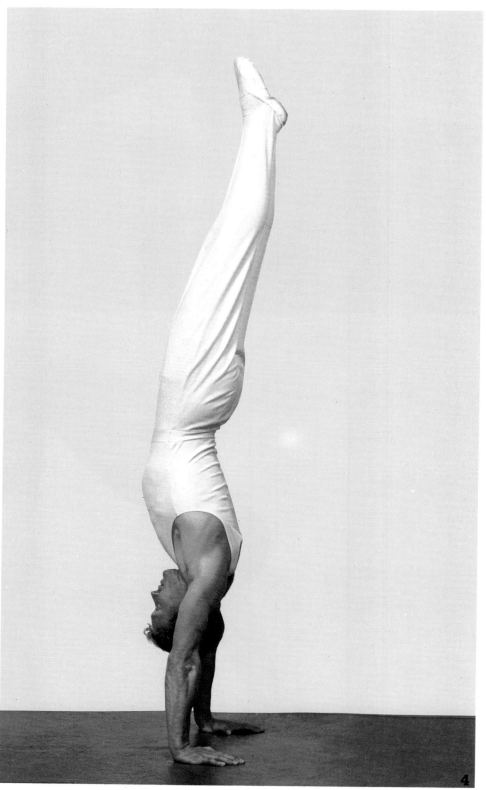

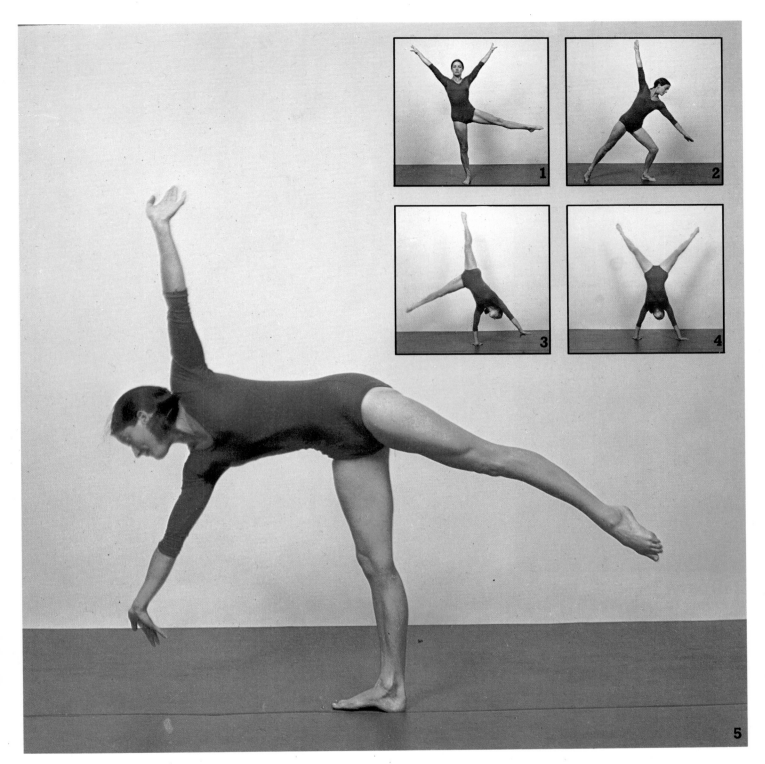

CARTWHEEL

As the name suggests, this move-ment resembles a revolving four-spoked wheel. The exercise shown is a left-handed cartwheel; another version can also be done to the right. Practise this exercise until you are able to perform it in either direction.

1. Stand with your feet apart, body straight and your arms stretched upwards and outwards. Lift your left leg sideways without leaning to the right while con-tinuing to stretch.

2. Place your left leg on the floor and bend your knee. Lean over your left leg stretching your left arm towards the floor.
Place your left hand on the floor about eighteen inches from the left foot with your fingers pointing backwards.

3. Push off from your left leg, straightening it as it leaves the floor. Keep both legs straight and wide apart while in the air. Make sure your back is straight and your hips and shoulders are in line with your hands.

4. Continue to wheel until your right hand reaches the floor.

5. Bring your legs over your head lifting your left and then your right hand as the right leg comes to the floor. Make sure your arms, legs and torso are moving in a straight line, neither bending forwards nor backwards.
Push away with your right hand as your left hand stretches upwards over your head. Do not let your left hand come across the front of the body.
Finish with both your feet on the floor in the straddle stand with your body straight and your arms stretching upwards.

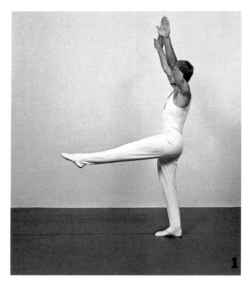

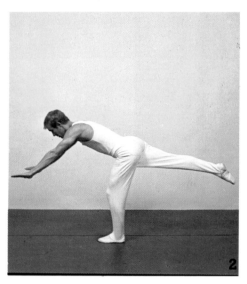

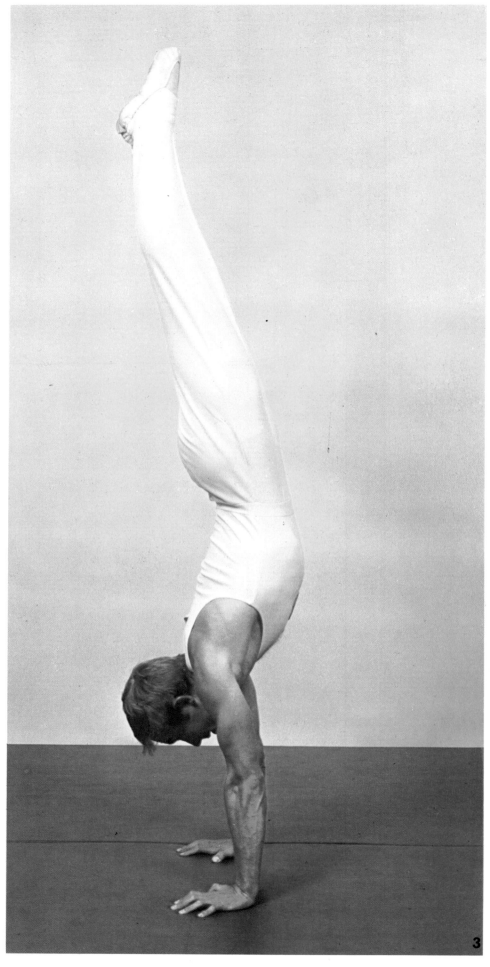

HANDSTAND

1. From a standing start, raise your arms above your head and lift one leg straight forwards.

2. Place your foot on the floor and tip forwards while slightly bending your knee. Stretch your other leg straight backwards and reach for the floor with your hands, placing them about twelve inches away from your foot.

Kick up into the handstand by pushing off from the foot which is on the floor and continuing to move the other leg upwards. Your arms should remain straight throughout.

3. Bring your two legs together and press them against each other. The tension of all your muscles is vital in order to maintain balance. Your shoulders and hips must be in line with your hands.

A second version of the handstand can be performed with your legs apart. Kick up into the handstand, allowing one leg to stretch over your head while the other counterbalances it on the other side.

CRAB

From the starting position, lie on your back, bend your knees and place your feet flat on the floor. Put your hands on the floor close to your shoulders with your arms bent and your fingers pointing towards your shoulders. Push upwards with your arms and legs and arch backwards. Push your shoulders directly above your hands without bending your arms. Pull your head between your arms.

This exercise helps increase suppleness. If you find it difficult, start with your legs bent, then progress to pushing the knees straight. It can also be useful having someone to help you when you first perform this exercise. Practise it as often as you can.

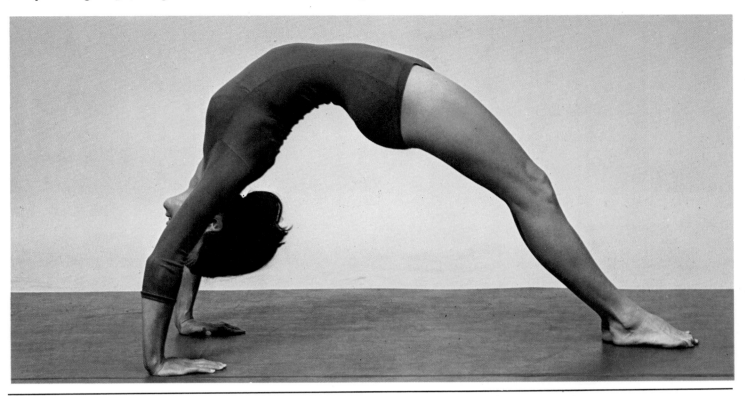

ONE-HANDED CARTWHEEL

1. From a standing start, lift your left leg to the side. Place your left hand on the floor about eighteen inches to the side of your left foot with your fingers pointing backwards. Keep your right arm and leg high. The leg on the floor may be bent or straight.
2. Push off from your left foot, swinging your right leg upwards. Hold your right arm up.
3. Continue the movement by swinging your legs over your head, using your left shoulder as a pivot. Keep your hips and legs in a straight line. Rotate over your left shoulder with your left arm locked out and your right arm out to the side or close to your body. Your body is now turning inwards and to the right.
4. Bring your right leg down to the floor and lift your left hand off the floor.

To finish, swing your right arm down and then up in front of your body, lifting your head and shoulders upwards. Move your left hand down and back. Bend your right leg and place your left leg behind your body.

This exercise should be executed in one smooth, circular motion.

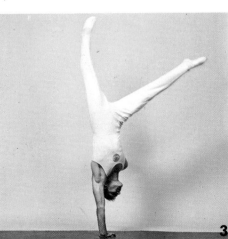

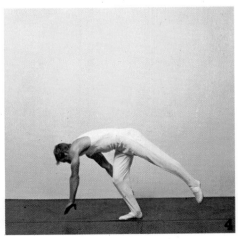

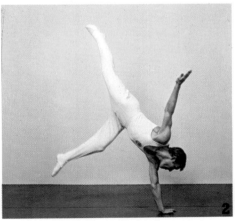

Gymnastics—4

This part of the gymnastics course shows you how to combine some of the movements you have already learned together with some new exercises to make a set, flowing routine. The routine is attractive to watch and much more exhilarating to perform than just repeating the movements on their own.

Go through each movement in isolation before attempting to combine them. Try to perfect each exercise, paying particular attention to the new movements: the leg circle and the splits.

To enable you to memorize the routine you might find it helpful to break it into three separate groups of exercises. Do this in any way that you find convenient. Practise them individually before combining them into the routine.

You will discover that to learn the routine will take more effort on your part than you had to make for other exercises in the gymnastics course. This is because a routine demands great concentration and co-ordination—not only when you are learning it but even when you are familiar with it.

You will also need more space to perform the routine than you do for the individual exercises. Practise outside, in a garden or a park, if you do not have enough room at home or in the gymnasium where you usually train.

When you have gone through the routine just once you will realize how worthwhile and satisfying your efforts have been. This satisfaction will not only be enjoyed by you but also by any of your friends who might be watching. Display gymnastics is becoming a popular sport.

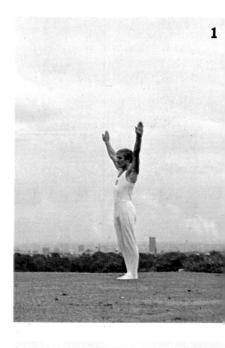

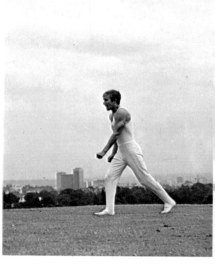

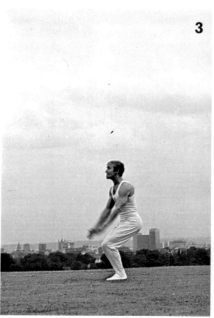

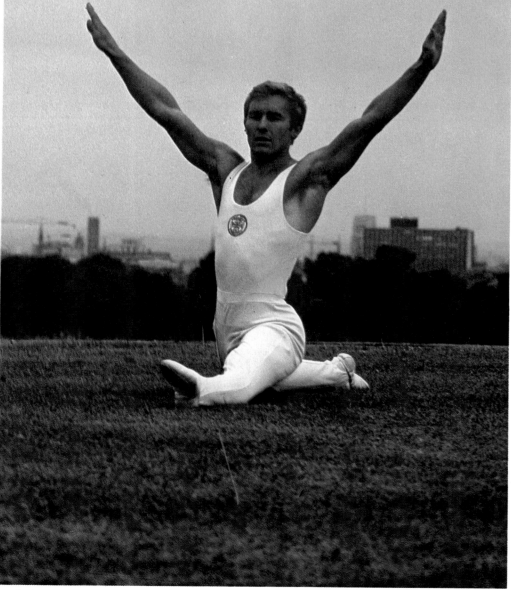

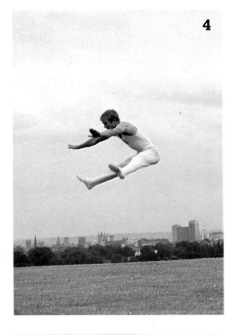

4

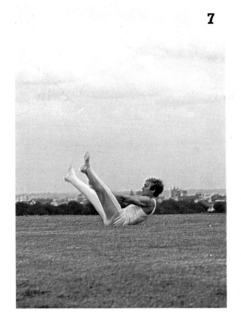

7

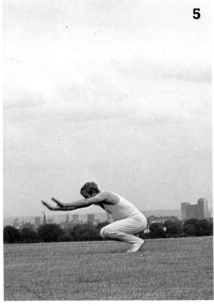

5

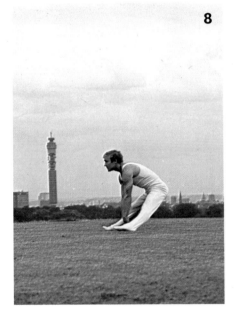

8

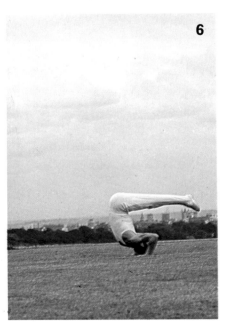

6

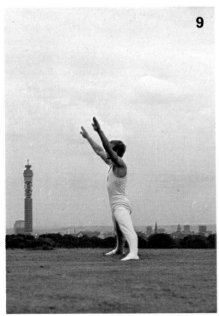

9

1. Take up the starting position with your feet together, body muscles tense and your arms raised above your shoulders. Pause for a few seconds and concentrate your attention on the movements that you are about to perform.
2. Take a few paces forwards.
3. Jump upwards from a two-foot take-off for a piked straddle jump.
4. Straddle your legs in the air, keeping them straight and as near horizontal as possible. Stretch your arms out towards your toes. Keep your back straight and your fingers and toes pointed.
5. Land on both feet with your legs together, knees bent and your arms pointing forwards.
6. Place your hands on the ground well in front of your body ready for the forward roll to straddle. Push from your toes, keeping your legs together. With your head tucked into your chest, roll onto your shoulders. Keep both your legs straight as your feet leave the ground.
7. Roll along your back with your legs straight and close to your body. Straddle your legs.
8. Bring your hands to the ground between your legs and as close as possible to your body. Looking straight ahead, press down on your hands and lean forwards until your hips are in line with your body.
9. Bring your body upright with your legs straight and apart, your arms stretched upwards, fingers pointed and your eyes looking straight ahead.

ROUTINE FOR WOMEN

From the starting position, step forwards into a scissor jump. Land on one leg. Step forwards into an arabesque. Tip into a forward roll. Immediately spring upwards making a half turn in the air. Land on both feet, bending your body for a backward roll. Kneel and place your hands on the ground for a headstand. Straddle your legs. Tip into a forward roll and make a quarter turn to kneeling, arms lifted. Stand and turn to the starting position. Cartwheel and immediately step into a handstand. Make a forward roll into a sitting straddle with arms raised. Turn in a side circle roll to the front support position. Spring upwards into a hollow straddle jump. Land with feet together, body upright.

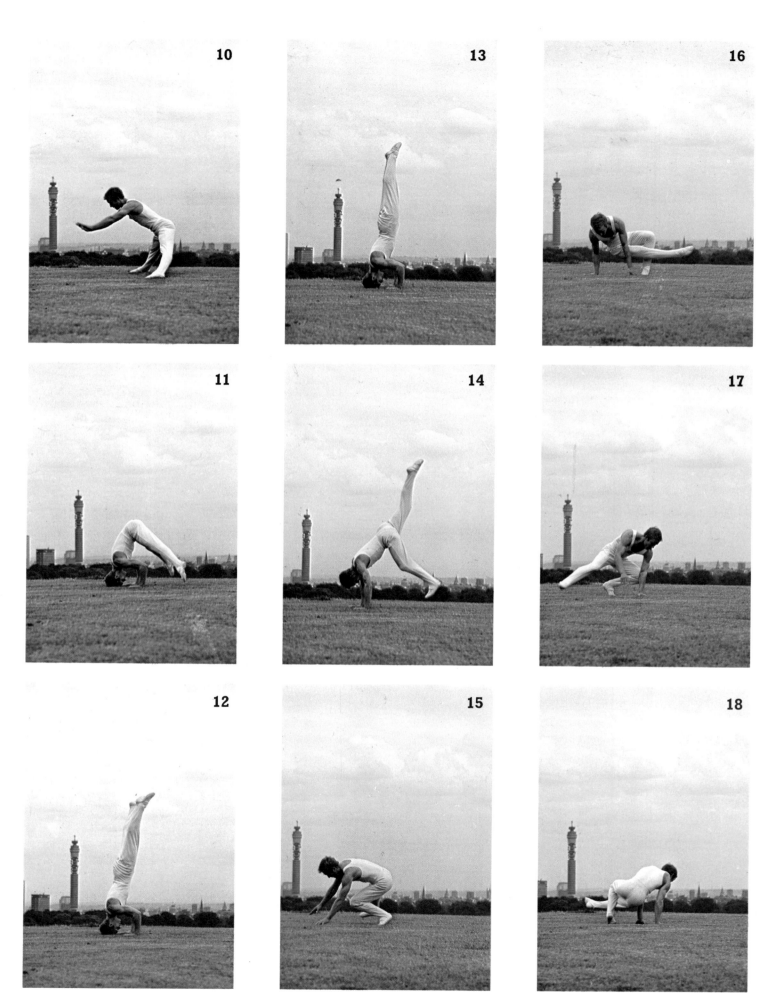

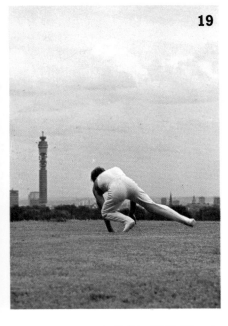

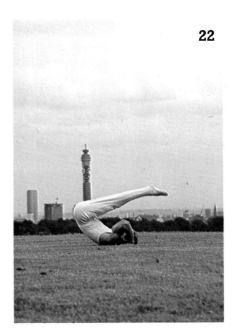

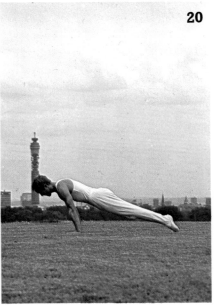

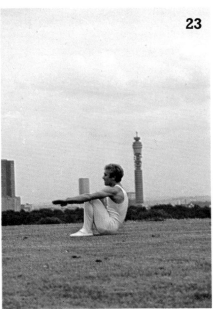

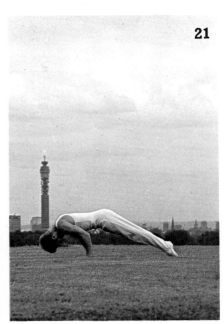

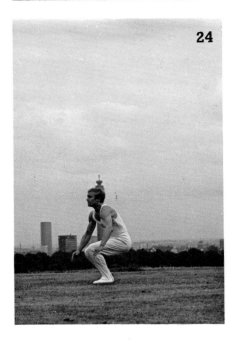

10. Bend your body sharply forwards from the hips for the headstand. Keep your arms straight and extended in front of your body. Point your fingers.

11. Place your hands on the ground in front of you. Put your head on the ground between your hands. Balance and bring your legs upwards, keeping them straight and apart with your toes pointed.

12. Raise your legs upwards, keeping them straight, until they are in line with your shoulders.

13. Bring your legs together. Balance on your hands and head.

14. Come down from the headstand bringing your left leg to the ground first. At the same time, raise your head from the ground and straighten your arms.

15. Swing your right leg in front of your body to begin a leg circle. Raise your hands off the ground to allow your leg to pass underneath.

16. Replace your hands on the ground immediately after your right leg has passed in front of your body. At the same time rotate your body in a quarter turn. This movement should be performed swiftly and smoothly and can be done using either your right or your left leg as a pivot.

17. As your right leg reaches your left leg hop upwards so that your right leg can pass under your body. Immediately replace your left leg on the ground and continue circling your right leg and body. Raise your hands again to allow your right leg to pass under your body, at the same time making a quarter turn.

18. Continue this turning movement, rotating your body and your right leg. Raise your hands and hop with your left leg to allow your right leg to pass under.

19. Stop rotating when your hands reach the position in which you started the leg circle.

20. Extend both legs backwards, supporting your body with your arms. Your toes are pointed and your head, body and legs are in a straight line.

21. Pull your legs forwards, bend your arms and tuck your head into your chest for a forward roll.

22. Tip forwards and roll onto your shoulders, keeping both your legs straight as your feet leave the ground.

23. Bend your legs as your head and shoulders come upwards. Place your feet flat on the ground with your arms stretched forwards and your fingers pointed.

24. Immediately spring upwards from both feet, turning your body at the same time.

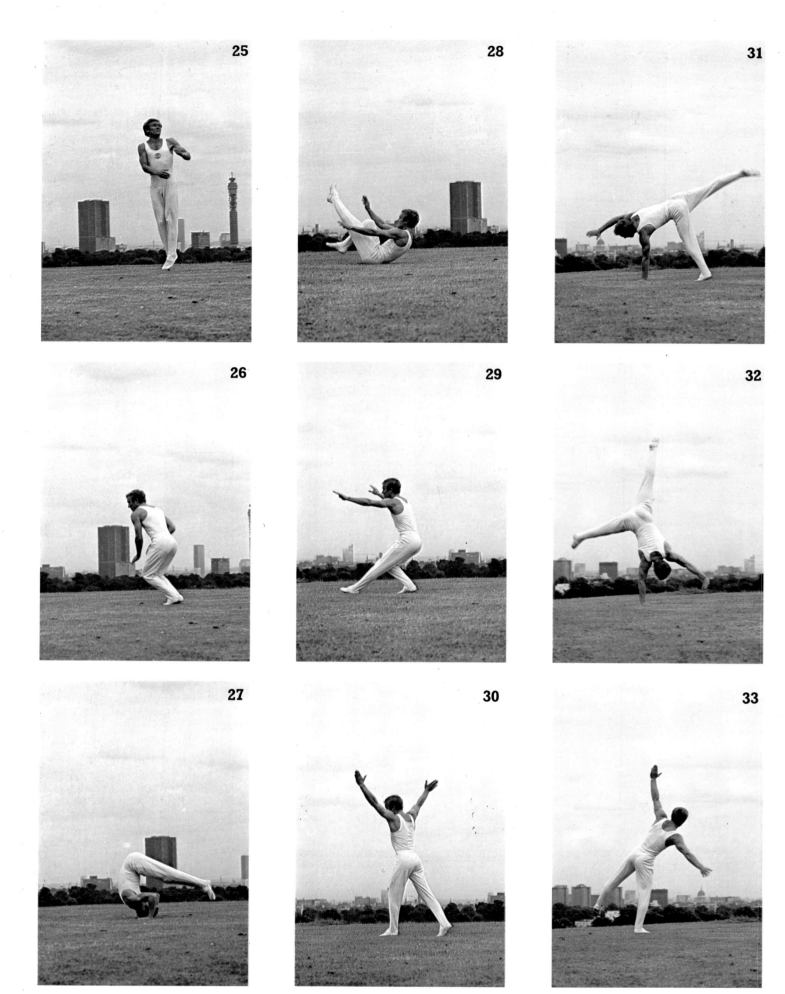

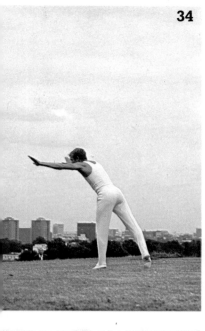

34

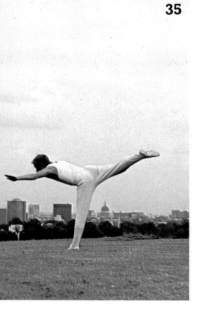

35

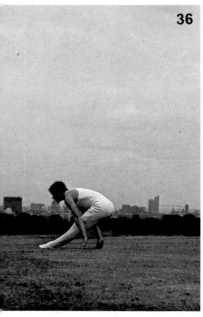

36

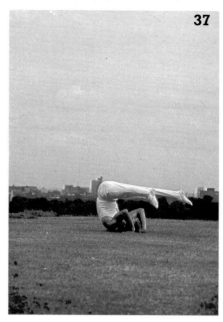

37

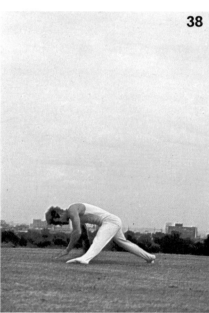

38

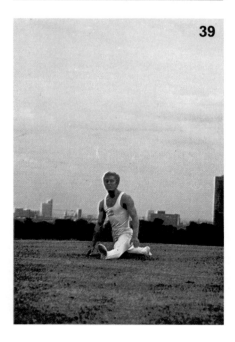

39

25. Continue twisting your body in the air, keeping your legs straight.

26. Twist round in a full circle, landing with your feet pointing in the same direction in which they were when you started to jump.

27. Place your hands on the ground in front of your body and tip down into a forward roll. Keep your head tucked into your chest and your legs straight.

28. Come up from the forward roll with your left leg stretched forwards and your right leg flat on the ground.

29. Stand up, with your left leg supporting your weight. Keep your arms stretched forwards, with your fingers pointed.

30. Lift your arms upwards and place your weight on your left foot to begin a cartwheel.

31. Bring your left hand to the ground. At the same time kick your right leg upwards, keeping it straight and your toes pointed. Pivot on your left shoulder.

32. Bring your legs over your body, keeping them straight and apart. Your legs, torso, head and arms should be moving smoothly and in one plane. Your left arm is now raised off the ground.

33. To finish the cartwheel, bring your right foot to the ground, following with your left. Keep your arms straight and raised above your shoulders.

34. Place your weight on your left foot. Keep your arms stretched forwards, and raise your right leg behind your body to come into an arabesque.

35. Keep your right leg straight and raise it as high as you can without straining. Stretch your arms to the side with your fingers pointed. Hold your head up and tense all your muscles. Your hips should be facing forwards.

36. Bring your right foot down to the ground. Place both hands behind your feet, keeping both legs straight, ready to perform a backwards roll.

37. Roll back onto your shoulders keeping your legs straight and apart and your toes pointed.

38. Continue moving your body over until your feet touch the ground. Begin turning your body to the left.

39. Continue turning your body to the left and slide your legs apart into the splits. Your legs should be straight and your toes pointed. Finish by lifting your arms upwards and to the side with your fingers pointed. Your body should be balanced in an upright position with your head up and eyes looking straight ahead.

Exercises for Stamina–1

Fitness has no limits. There are always some means by which you can improve even further the physical prowess and natural agility of your body. And fitness is the surest indication that you are in the best of health—able to enjoy life to the full, with zest and stamina.

Whether you are a keen follower of sport, a budding adept at yoga or have been doing some form of exercise programme, your general stamina can be built up even more through this course of strength and endurance exercises. Over a period of time you can learn to exert yourself without becoming breathless and to recover quickly from any physical activity which taxes your energy. The development of this kind of power fitness is brought about only by a series of dynamic movements—the range of movements which this course is designed to give you.

These exercises provide you with untiring, vigorous energy. They demand unflinching effort and determination on your part, especially as the number of repetitions of each exercise increases. For this reason you can only start the course if you have reached a reasonable level of fitness through following a particular sport or by practising a daily set of exercises of some kind.

In two parts, *Exercises for Stamina* enables you to aim for the pinnacle of fitness so that you become healthier and more energetic. Your heart, lungs and circulatory system are heavily involved when doing the exercises which also demand muscular endurance.

Your heart and lungs have to work increasingly harder as the course progresses. This is a unique aspect of the exercises and the benefits which it brings to your health could have far-reaching affects.

All of the exercises have been selected to build up your strength and endurance. Strength is the muscular ability to overcome maximum resistance once or greater resistance a few times. The exercises provide this resistance. The quality of endurance is something different. It is the ability to work or exercise hard for long periods of time and to recover quickly from fatigue.

This course is, therefore, designed to be vigorous. It demands effort and determination if you are to achieve worthwhile results. The exercises are a subtle combination, increasing your strength while at the same time gradually building up your level of endurance through the number of repetitions. After a period of persistent exercises you are rewarded for your efforts with a tough fitness suitable for a wide range of physical activity. Your body will have far more muscular power than the average person's and your level of endurance will enable you to participate in long periods of continuous physical effort without getting tired.

And the course greatly improves your breathing so that you inhale and exhale deeply and economically—with control and in a way which ensures vital and energizing lungs.

The first section of the course consists of exercises which activate all the major muscles in your body against part or the whole of your body weight. This develops your strength. The number of repetitions for each exercise improves your level of muscular and general endurance. The minimum number of repetitions are only a guide and should be reduced or increased to suit your level of fitness. Begin with a number of repetitions which are not too easy for you but which at the same time do not strain you or even cause you some physical damage.

The second part of the course provides you with a number of exercises requiring the use of small weights so that you become even fitter and learn to control speed and mobility.

The rest pauses between each exercise are an important part of the whole course. These should gradually be reduced so that you can go from one exercise to another as quickly as possible in order to keep your pulse rate high. Your pulse rate is an indicator which tells you just how hard your heart and lungs are working and provides you with a means to check your progress.

This course enables you to reach a peak of fitness entirely at your own pace. It is up to your own judgement when and how far to increase the number of repetitions. Because of this the course is adaptable, suiting all levels of fitness. It enables you to first find out just which level of effort is comfortable for you and then provides you with the means to increase your strength and endurance. The benefits to your health last for a long time.

And the exercises are varied to give you enjoyment and a wide range of movements for your limbs and all the major muscles in your body.

Resolve to start this course and gain the vitalizing benefits of a strong heart, healthy lungs, good breathing and a level of fitness which not only makes you feel good but gives vigour to your personality and looks.

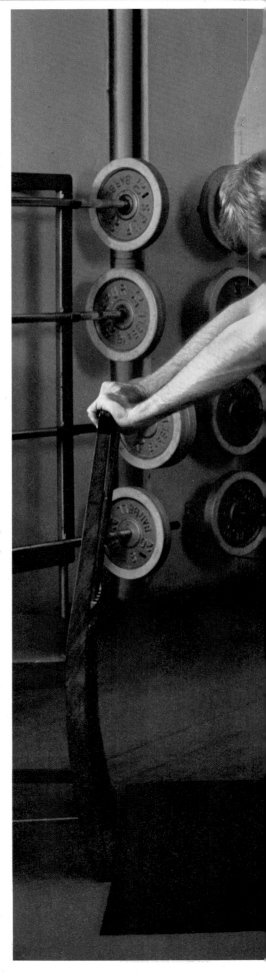

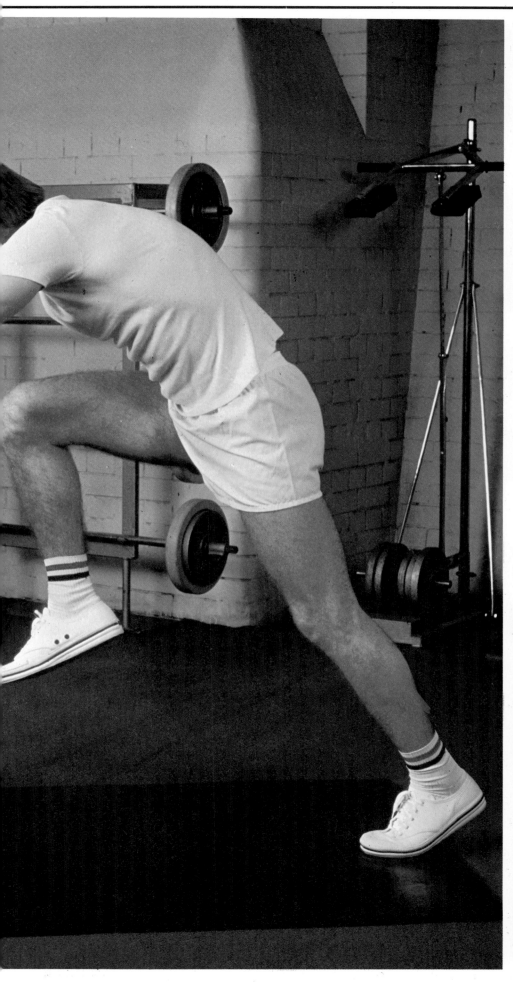

ANGLE RUNNING/left
Stimulates the heart, improves the circulation, limbers up the legs and abdominal muscles

Place your hands on the back of a strong chair. Keep your feet slightly apart and lean your body at an angle of 45°.
Alternately raise the thighs close to your chest in a running action. Raise your thighs as high as they will reach each time.
Always land on your toes. This makes the movement easier and more flowing.
Keep your neck fairly straight and don't stare down at your knees. Breathe freely.
Begin with 15 repetitions. Count a repetition each time your left thigh touches your chest.
Gradually work up to 30 repetitions.

V SITS/below
Strengthens the abdominal muscles, slims the waist, aids circulation, stimulates the heart and improves breathing

Lie on your back with your feet together. Keep your hands and arms on the floor behind your head. Raise your legs and trunk with a swing until your hands touch your feet and you are balanced on the buttocks. Try to control your balance throughout.
Breathe in as you fold up and out as you return to the starting position.
Begin with 15 repetitions and aim to reach 30 repetitions or more if you can.

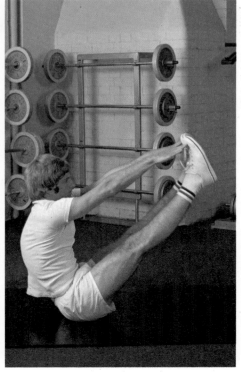

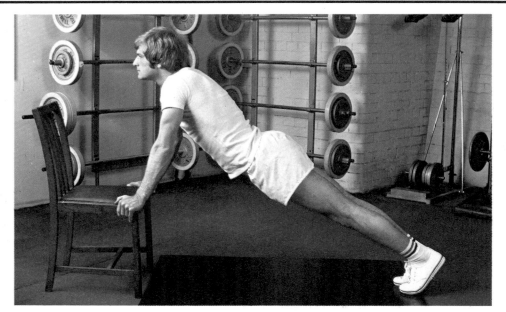

ARMS HIGH PRESS UP/left
Strengthens the chest, shoulder and arm muscles, keeps the pulse rate high, helps to control breathing

Place both hands on a sturdy chair, toes on floor and feet shoulder-width apart. Keep your body straight.
While keeping the body straight, bend your elbows bringing your chest close to the chair. Then extend your arms again.
Breathe in as you press up and out as you lower to the chair. Begin at 15 repetitions and work up to 30 repetitions or more.

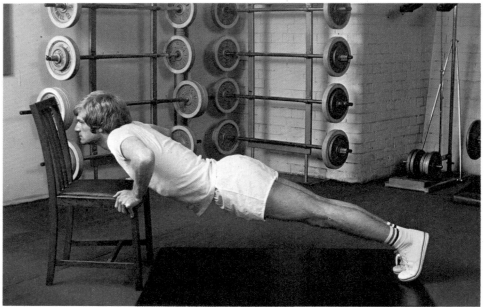

Some of the exercises in this course are easier than others. This is by design in order to permit the pulse rate to slow down and lower slightly.
So if you find an exercise just that little less difficult than another don't try to force the pace. It is intended as a kind of breather so that you can do the next exercise with that much more vigour and energy. When doing the less difficult exercises make a conscious effort to relax.

WIDE ARM PULL UPS/right
Strengthens the arm, shoulder and upper back muscles, keeps the pulse rate high, helps to control breathing

Place two sturdy chairs about three feet apart. Place a strong broom-stick between the chairs with the ends of the handle well on to the chairs.
Now lie on the floor with your shoulders directly below the broomstick.
Grip the broomstick at both ends with your palms facing towards your chest.
Keep your body straight and heels on the floor as you pull yourself upwards until your chest touches the broomstick. Then lower yourself into your original position. Breathe in as you rise and out as you lower.
Work from 10 to 30 repetitions.

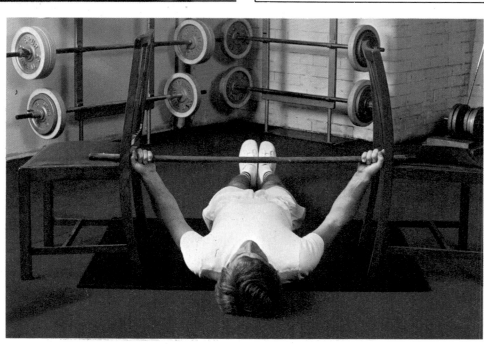

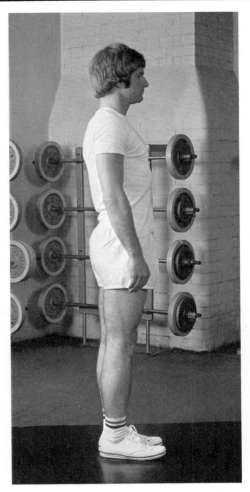

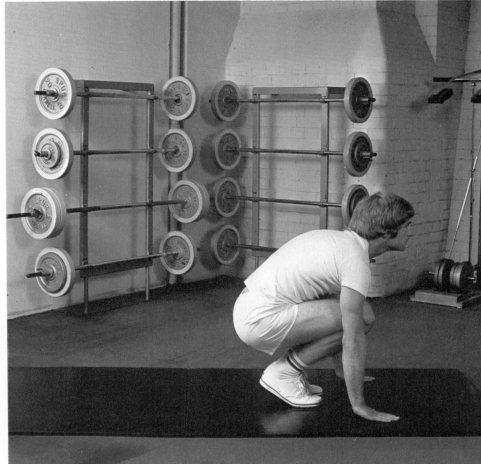

BURPEES
Keeps the pulse rate high and exercises the legs, strengthens the arm, shoulder and abdominal muscles

Stand in a normal standing position, arms by your sides and feet placed together. Keep your head straight and look in front of you. Bend both knees until you can place your hands on the floor just outside your legs and close to your feet. Now jump backwards so that your body is straight and you are supported by your arms. Return to the starting position through the middle position. Breathe freely throughout. Begin with 15 repetitions and gradually progress to 30 or 40.

When you complete this exercise do some on-the-spot running. Do not lift the knees high. Try to be as relaxed as you can. Breathe freely throughout. Run for 30 repetitions. Count a repetition each time your left foot touches the floor. Do not over-exert yourself when doing this exercise. It is intended to exercise your leg muscles gently. So try to be as relaxed as you can even as the repetitions increase.

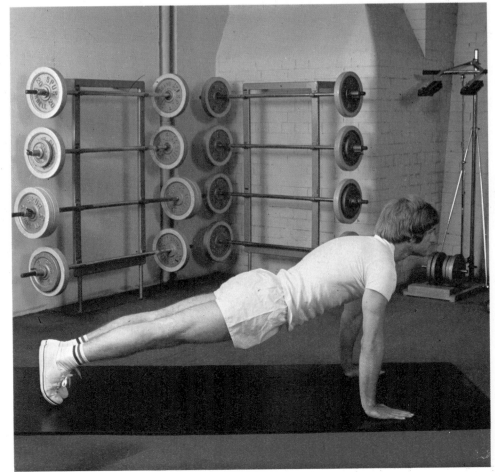

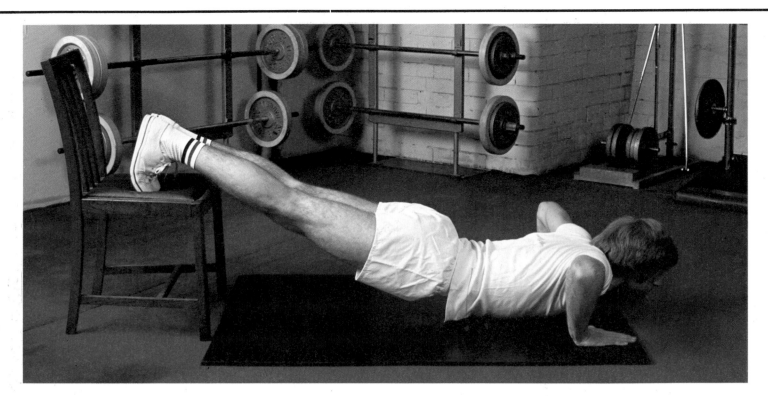

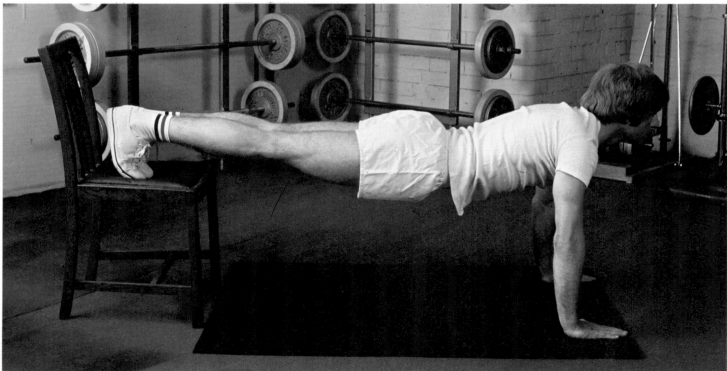

FEET HIGH PRESS UP
Strengthens the chest, shoulder and arm muscles, helps to keep the pulse rate high, improves breathing

Place both feet on a sturdy chair. Place your hands on the floor shoulder-width apart. Keep your body straight and your arms extended.
Then bend your elbows and lower your chest. Go as low as you can without being too uncomfortable. Breathe in as you press up and out as you lower to the floor. Start at 15 repetitions and work up to 30 repetitions or more. If you have difficulty aiming for 15 repetitions lower the number to 10 and gradually progress upwards until you reach 15, 20, 25, 30 and more. This exercise is one of the best endurance exercises involving strength. Without exerting yourself too much always try to increase the number of repetitions. You'll find that this becomes easier and easier each session until you can do more without discomfort.

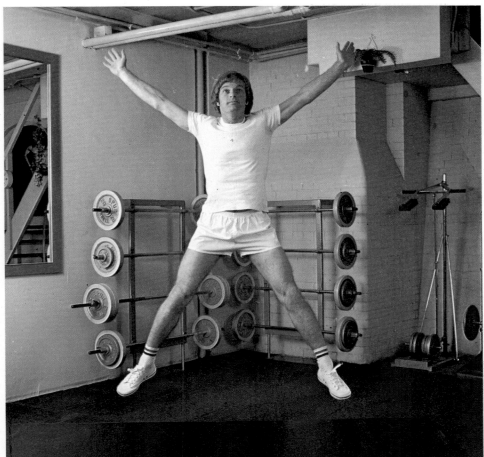

STAR JUMPS
Develops spring and power in the legs, keeps the pulse rate high, strengthens the calf muscles

Take up a normal standing position with your feet a few inches apart. Bend both knees to lower your body. Leap high in the air and spread your legs and arms into the Star position. Bend both knees to take the shock of landing.
Consciously stretch your legs and arms as much as possible when you jump, keeping them straight. Don't bend your neck and out-stretch your fingers.
Breathe freely throughout.
Begin with 10 leaps and work up to 20 or 30 leaps.

When you have gone through your optimum of repetitions begin running on the spot. Remember to do this in a relaxed way, never lifting the knees high.
Run for 30 repetitions, counting a repetition each time your left foot touches the floor.
Running on the spot in this way is intended to slow down your pulse rate slightly before you go on to the exercise which completes the first half of the stamina-exercise course.

LEAP TO HIGH CROUCH
Develops power in the legs and abdominal muscles, stimulates the heart, improves the capacity of the lungs, aids circulation and helps reactions

Take a normal standing position with feet almost together. Leap upwards, tucking your knees in close to your chin.
Land on your toes and do two low skip jumps then repeat the leap to high crouch.
Breathe freely throughout.
Begin with six repetitions and work up to 10 or 12 full jumps. Increase this number if you feel you can.

The number of repetitions given at the end of each exercise are stipulated by an expert. Pay attention to them and don't try to do too much at first. You could over-strain yourself and possibly even do some damage. Start at the lowest number of repetitions and gradually work upwards. Never start at the highest number of repetitions no matter how enthusiastic you are. You'll eventually reach the maximum number.

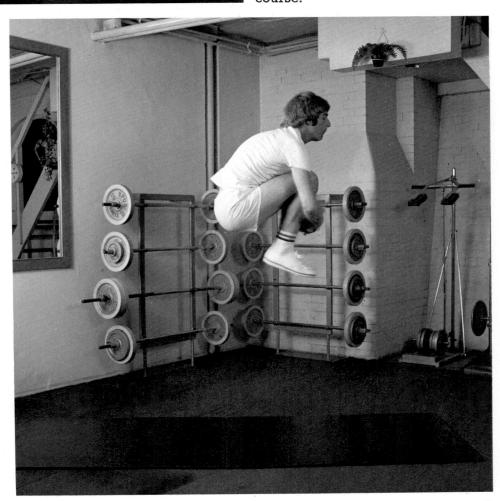

147

Exercises for Stamina—2

These exercises, the second part of the stamina course, are designed to make you even fitter—more energetic and healthier. They improve still further the efficiency of your heart and lungs, your powers of endurance and strength and your overall fitness.

By following the first half of the course you should have reached a reasonable level of fitness, able to call upon increased resources of strength and endurance. The first set of exercises, while compact in themselves, are also intended as a preparation for exercises involving the use of weights.

Contrary to popular misconception, weights are not intended merely to build up muscles. If you follow these exercises you will find that, used with care, they tone you up without making you muscle-bound. And you can progress if you wish to our complete weight training course.

By using weights you have to work against a given resistance to the number of repetitions which you can comfortably cope with. This calls upon extra effort from your heart and lungs, greatly im-proving your stamina capabilities much more quickly than weight-less exercises do—provided you use them consistently every day.

Weights are also adaptable. When you have completed this course of exercises the 20-pound weights can be made heavier to give you greater resistance and an opportunity to become even stronger and with more endurance capability.

To gain the maximum benefits from these exercises and to build upon the fitness achieved in the first part of the course requires some degree of dedica-tion. Practise them every day. If you begin to miss days your progress will be slowed down. Setting aside a special time to do the exercises each day helps to guarantee that you won't forget to do them.

To cope with the stresses and tensions of everyday life requires a good level of fitness. This course of exercises provides you with that fitness, and more. Resolve to start the course and you'll soon dis-cover in yourself a new zest for life and renewed health and vigour.

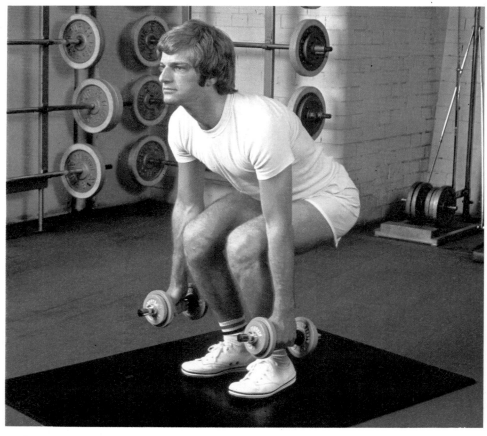

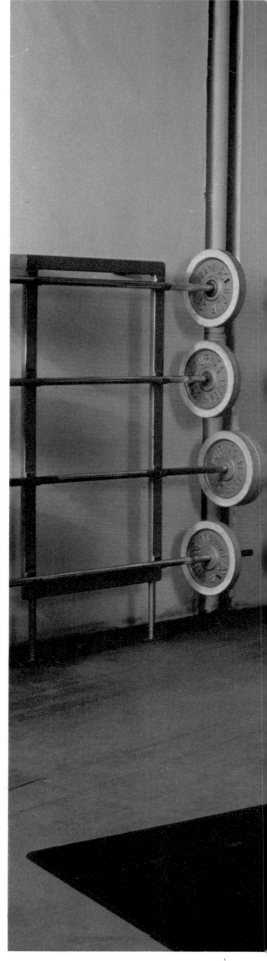

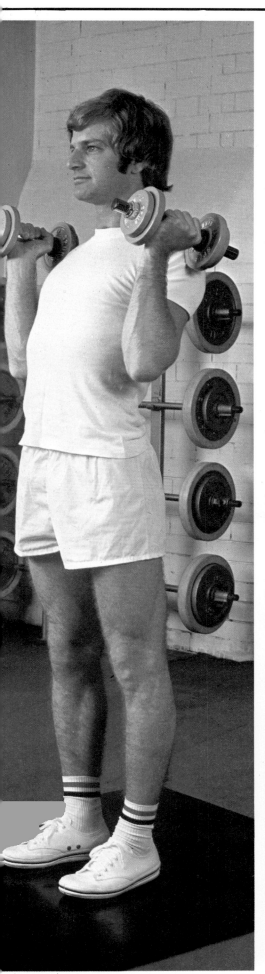

POWER CLEAN/left
Develops all-round muscular power, stimulates the heart and aids the circulation

Stand between two dumb-bells with your feet approximately 10 inches apart. Bend your knees to right angles. Lean forward keeping your back flat.
Grip each dumb-bell with your hands, knuckles facing outwards. Straighten your legs, hips and back, bending your elbows as the dumb-bells pass your thighs in order to bring each dumb-bell to shoulder level. Carry out this action briskly from the floor to your shoulders. Breathe in as you pull upwards and out as you return to the starting position.
The dumb-bells should weigh about 20 pounds each.
Work from 15 to 30 repetitions.

SIDE BENDS/below
Strengthens the muscles on each side of the spine and waist, improves mobility and helps to slim the abdomen

Stand with your feet astride. Hold one dumb-bell in your left hand and place your free hand around the side of your neck. Bend slightly so that the dumb-bell is level with your left knee. Bend to your side away from the dumb-bell and then bend back to the starting position. Repeat with the dumb-bell in your right hand. Keep your back as straight as possible and make sure that your head is held erect. Breathe freely throughout.
The dumb-bell should weigh about 20 pounds.
Begin with 15 repetitions to each side and progress to 25 repetitions or more.

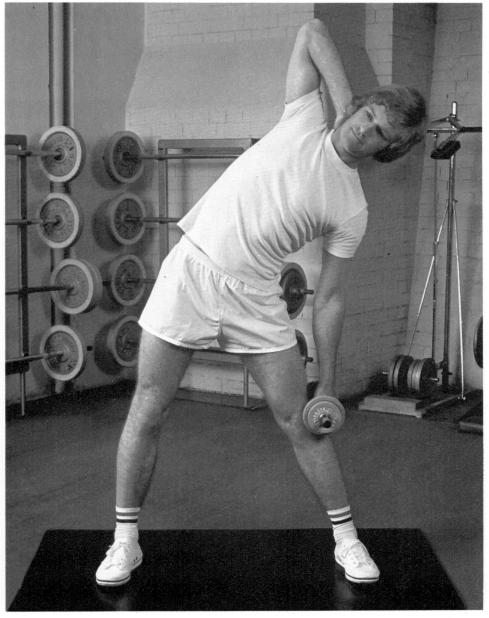

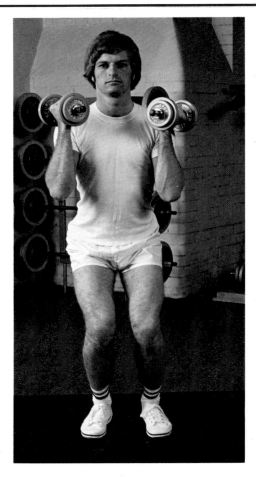

HEAVE PRESS
Develops the power of the upper body, tones the stomach and arm muscles and improves the sense of balance

Stand between two dumb-bells with your feet approximately 10 inches apart. Bend your knees to right angles. Keep your back flat but not vertical.

Grip each dumb-bell with your knuckles facing outwards.

Bend both knees slightly and heave the two dumb-bells to shoulder level. Then heave them above your head so that your arms are straight and outstretched.

Breathe in as you heave upwards and out as you lower the dumb-bells back to your shoulders.

The dumb-bells should weigh about 20 pounds each.

Begin at 15 repetitions and progress to 30 or more.

Increase the number of your repetitions gradually. Don't force the pace until you are absolutely sure that you can reasonably cope with the extra strain on your muscles, heart and lungs. If you try too much too soon there is the danger that you might do some damage.

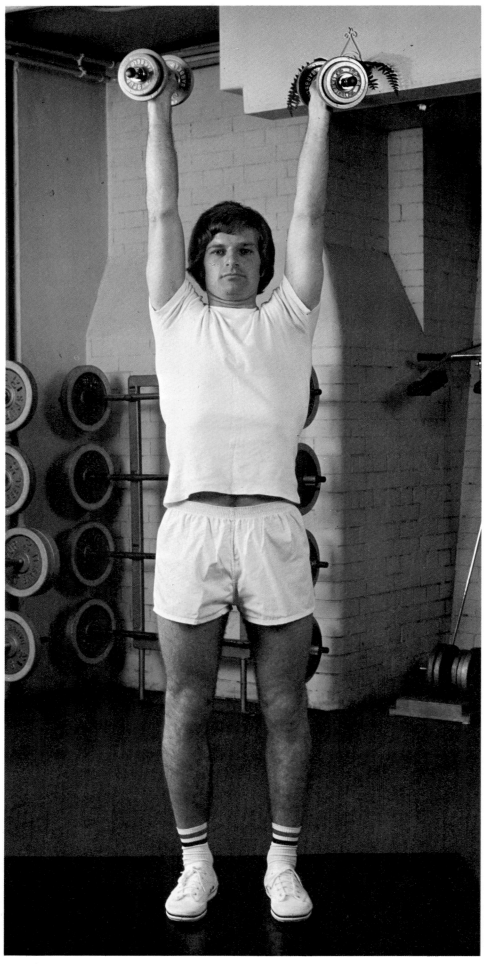

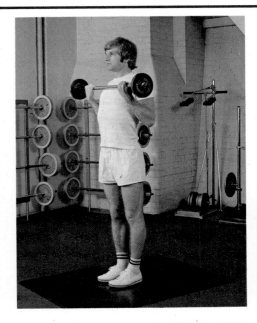

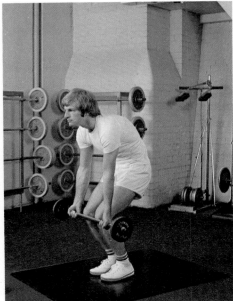

VERTICAL LEAPS/below
Develops drive and spring in the legs, improves the sense of balance, strengthens the neck muscles and tones up the waist and calf muscles

Stand with your feet about 10 inches apart. Hold the bar-bell across the shoulders and behind the head. Make sure that your shoulders are held well back. Drive upwards by extending both legs. Aim for as much height as you can reach. Land on your toes and bend both knees quickly to lessen the impact of landing. Breathe freely throughout the exercise. The bar-bell should weigh about 20 pounds.
Begin with 10 jumps and progress to 30 or more jumps.

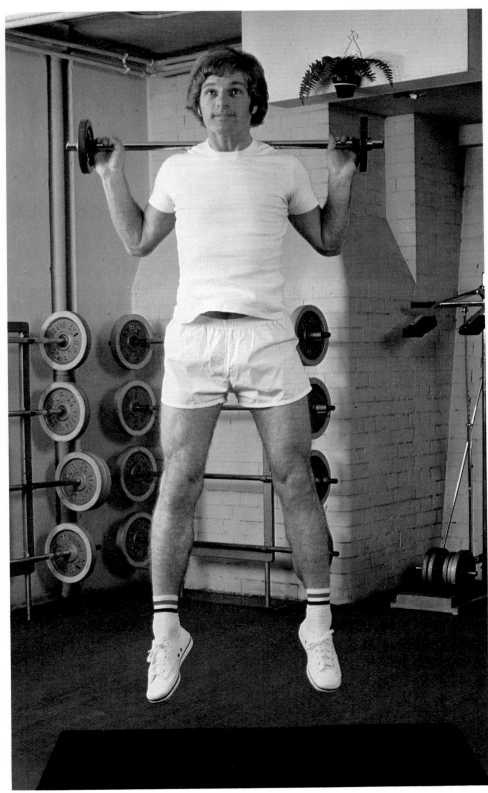

ROUND BACK CURLS/above
Exercises the spinal, upper back and arm muscles

Grasp a bar-bell keeping your hands about 10 inches apart and your palms facing forwards. Your arms should be straight, your knees and back bent. The bar-bell should be brought level with your knees. Vigorously extend your legs and back as you bend to bring the bar-bell to chest level. Keep the bar-bell close to your body throughout the exercise. Hold your body erect and expand your chest when you raise the bar-bell from your knees. Breathe in on the upward movement and out as you lower.
The bar-bell should weigh about 20 pounds.
Begin with 15 repetitions and work up to 30.

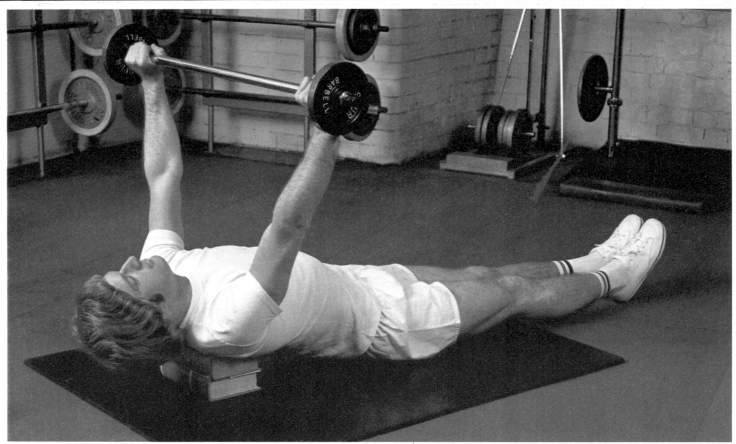

BENCH PRESS/above
Develops the arms, shoulders and chest and increases power in the forearms

Lie on your back on the floor. Prop your shoulders up by using one or two books. Grip the bar-bell across your chest with your hands about shoulder-width apart.
Press the bar-bell vertically upwards until your arms are straight. Return the bar-bell to your chest. Breathe in as the bar-bell goes up and out as you lower to chest. The bar-bell should weigh about 20 pounds.
Begin with 15 repetitions and increase to 25 repetitions.

STEP-UPS/right
Creates work for the lungs and heart, and exercises the legs

Place a bar-bell on your shoulders, well behind your head. Stand in front of a strong box, stool or low chair.
Step up on to the box with the left foot first and then the right foot. Continue this for half of the repetitions and then lead with the right foot for the second half. Breathe freely throughout.
The bar-bell should be 20 pounds. Begin at 20 step-ups and progress to 40 or 60.
Count one repetition each time you have both feet on the box.

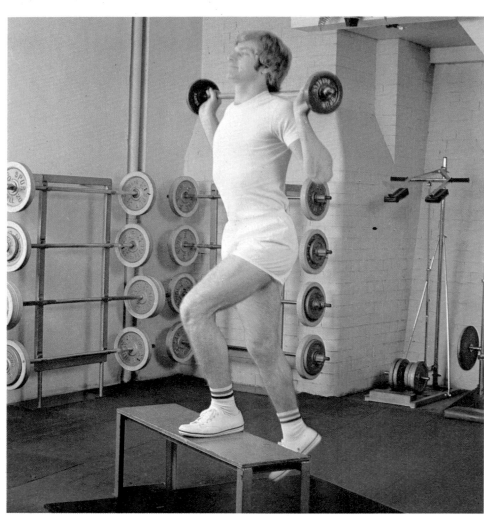

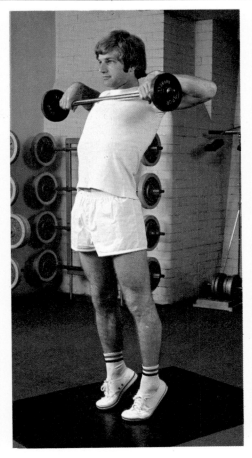

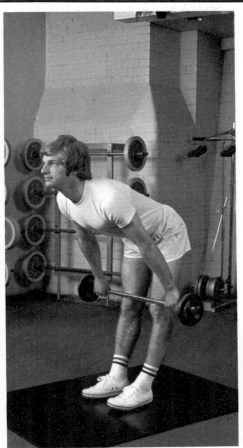

ROWING FROM KNEES/left
Strengthens the legs, back, arms and shoulders and keeps the pulse rate up

Grip the bar-bell with your hands shoulder-width apart and hold it at knee level. Keep your feet about 10 inches apart and your back flat, bending from the waist to 45°. Your knuckles should be facing forwards.
Pull the bar-bell almost chin high as you swing the hips forward into the arch position. Raise yourself on your toes and keep your chest and elbows high.
Breathe in as you pull and out as you return to the starting position. The bar-bell should weigh about 20 pounds.
Begin at 15 repetitions and progress to 30.

These exercises are designed to improve your strength and power of endurance. So don't take things too easy. Expend as much effort as you can without causing undue strain. Increase the repetitions when capable of even more stamina.

V SITS/right
Strengthens the abdominal and stomach muscles, slims the waist, aids circulation, stimulates the heart and improves breathing

Lie on your back with your feet together. Keep your hands and arms on the floor behind your head. Grip the dumb-bell with the weight centred in the middle.
Raise your legs and trunk with a swing until your hands touch your feet and you are balanced on the buttocks. Try to control your balance throughout.
Breathe in as you fold up and out as you return to the starting position. Begin with 15 repetitions and aim to reach 30 repetitions or more if you can.

To start this course you will need two 20-pound dumb-bells and a 20-pound bar-bell. You can buy these at any sports shop or hire them in most gymnasiums. Repeat the exercises once or twice to get used to the weights before beginning to increase the number of your repetitions. And don't start the course with heavier weights. Wait until you're stronger.

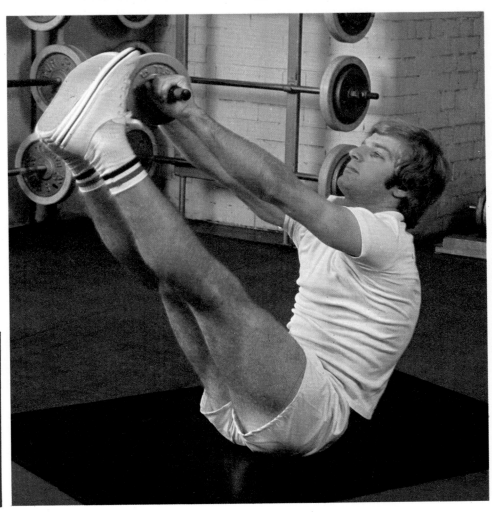

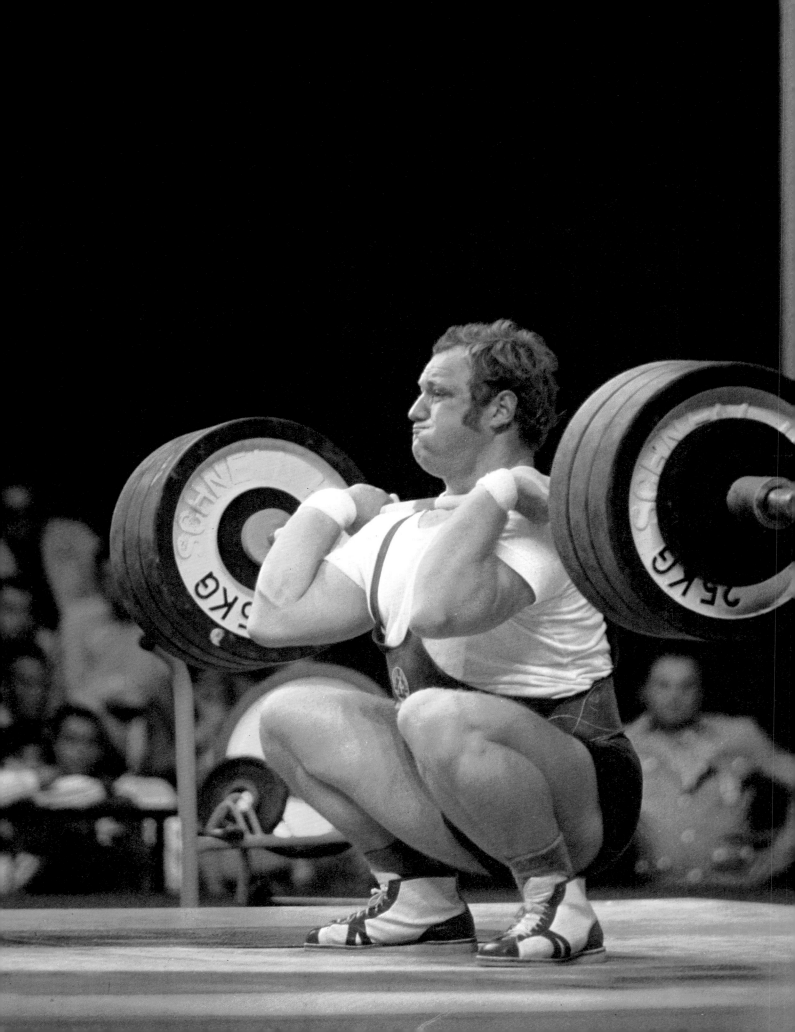

Weight Training for Strength— and Fitness

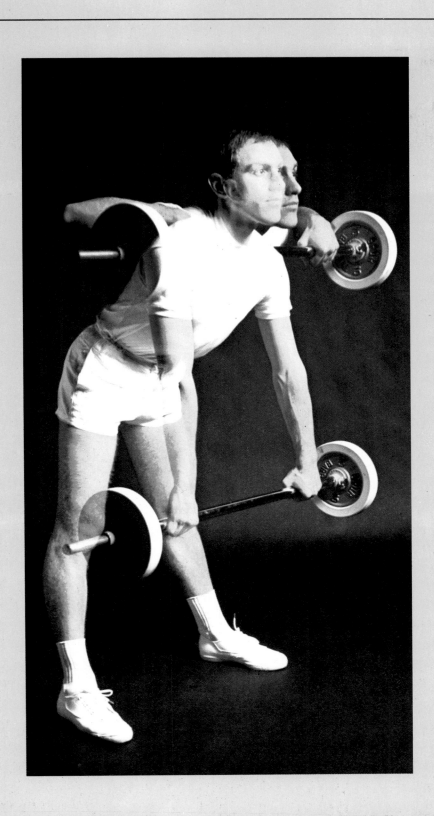

This is a complete short but comprehensive programme of weight–training for men – an easy-to-follow sequence of exercises which will increase your strength and improve your physique.

Weights, of course, are not merely muscle-builders. Used gently, they're not even primarily that. With a sensible approach you can use weights for improving your endurance, your suppleness, your heart-lung efficiency—your overall fitness.

Most young men at some time or another think about or take up a course of physique improvement. If they go about it in the right way, there's no doubt they'll get results, in terms of muscular growth, quite quickly. Massive muscular development is another matter, requiring complete dedication. This course is not concerned with that : it's designed to increase your fitness *and* your physique, but not necessarily making you into a muscle man. If you want, you can increase the weight and number of repetitions involved to start towards that goal.

Why use weights ?

The principle of muscle growth is the same whatever the aim. In weight training, the muscles are asked to work against a given resistance (weight) a given number of times each day. When the 'load' can be handled without undue effort, the resistance and or the number of repetitions are increased.

The great advantage of weights is their versatility and adaptability. You can adjust the weight and repetitions to suit you, and you can cover (and develop) all the major muscles in the body.

About this course

All you need to start are two 5lb or 10lb (2kg or 4kg) weights and a bar. Repeat the exercises once to start with until you see how they suit you, and then increase the repetitions as appropriate. Do each one five times and increase by one each day. Do not go straight into a heavy, strenuous session, and do not start with heavier weights. It's also advisable to go through some warm–up exercises first – you could practice isometrics and isotonics, for instance.

Breathe in on the upward movements. **1.** Starting position for all lifts : knees bent, arms and back straight, shoulders just in front of bar, eyes to front. **2.** Pull bar chin-high from start ; develops legs, hips, back, arms, shoulders. **3.** Palms forwards, bend and stretch arms ; develops muscles in front of upper arms. **4.** Bar on shoulders, press to arms' length ; develops shoulders, upper back, muscles at back of upper arms. **5.** Raise elbows sideways until bar touches top of chest ; develops upper back, shoulders, arms. **6.** Dumb-bell in one hand, bend from side to side, breathing freely ; develops muscles of spine, side of trunk. **7.** Rest bar on shoulders, bend knees ; develops legs, hips, chest, back. **8.** Lying on back press bar-bell upwards ; develops chest, shoulders, back of upper arms. **9.** Lift bar-bell from start close to body and on to chest ; develops legs, hips, back, arms. **10.** Start flat on floor, tilting board as fitness improves ; breathe out as you sit up ; develops waist-line muscles. **11.** Lying on bench, bar across thighs ; breathe in as bar is moved in half-circle to behind head, and out on return ; mobilizes chest walls, develops shoulders, chest.

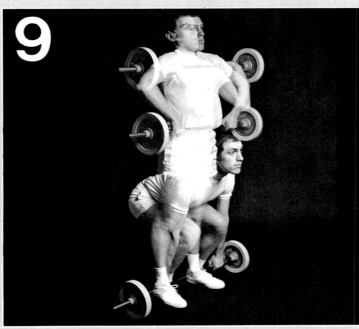

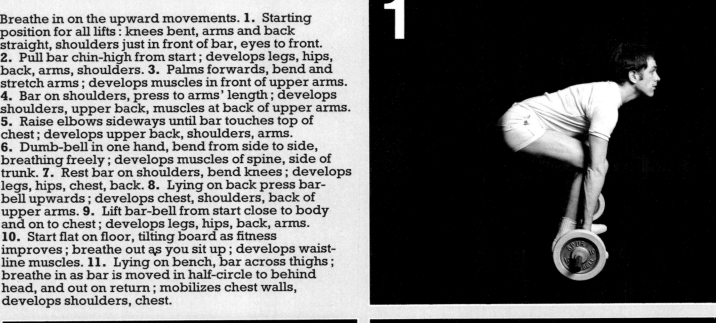

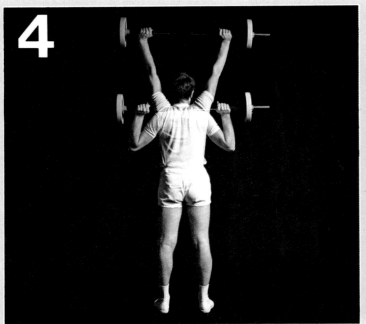

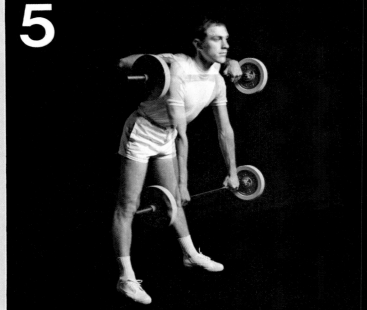

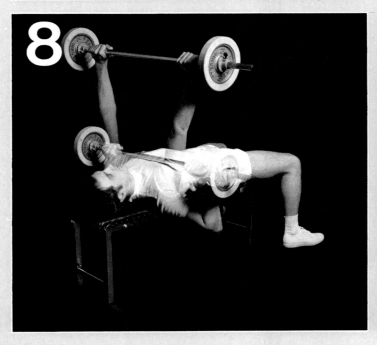

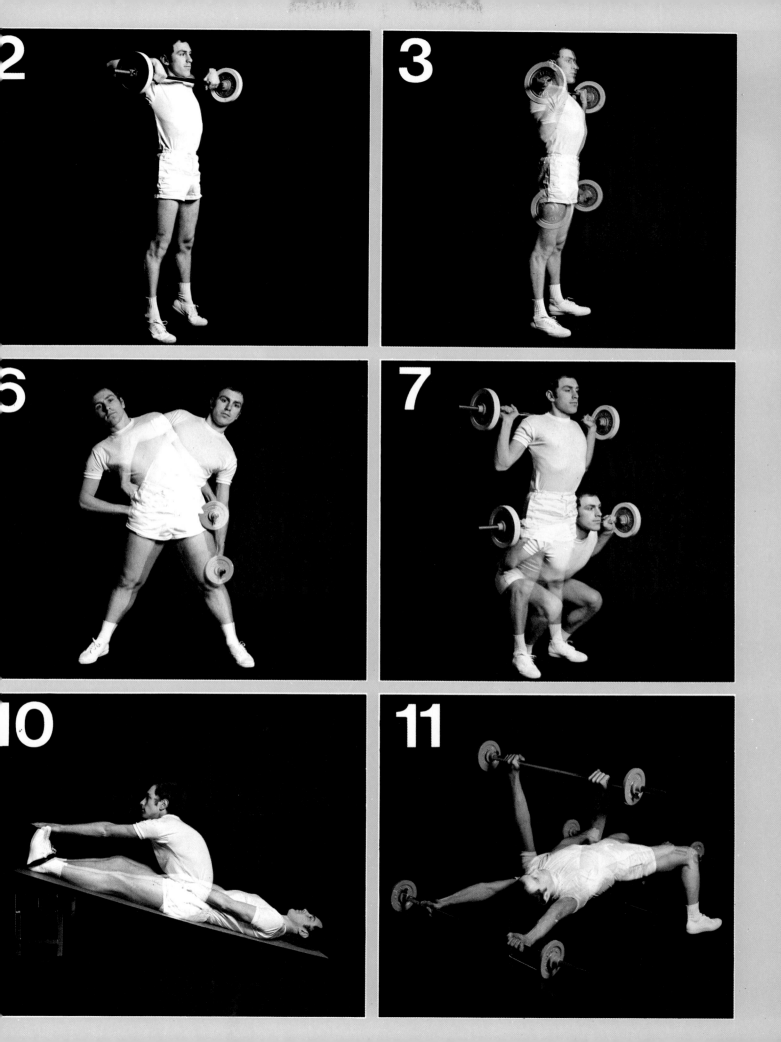

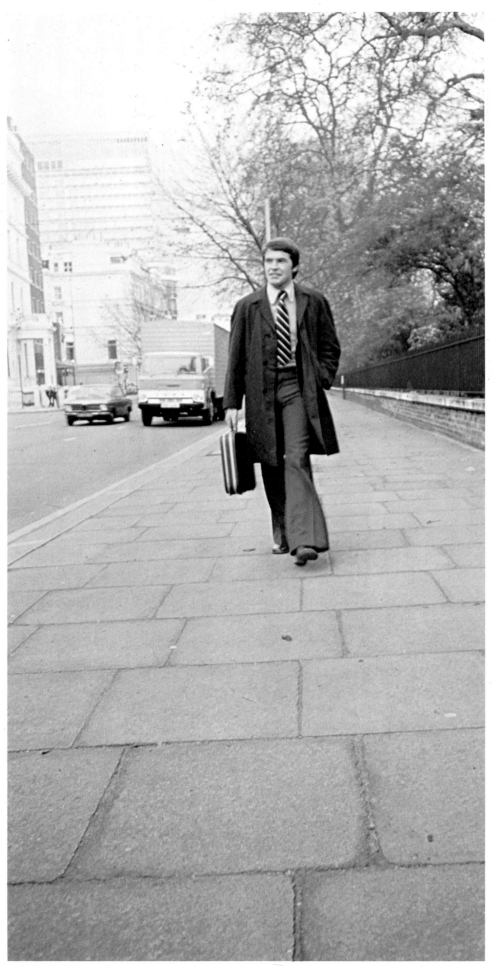

Rediscover

How often have you stood at a bus stop or sat in a traffic jam on the way to work and thought that there must be a better way of getting from place to place?

If you live in the suburbs of a big city and it takes you forty minutes during the rush hour to reach your place of work by bus or train, the chances are that you could walk the whole way in just over an hour, or less if you can work out a few short cuts through interesting side streets or across public parks or gardens.

As a general rule you can figure on no more than 50 per cent being added to the time it takes you to get from door to door when you walk to work instead of riding. And isn't walking more fun? Think of the time wasted in walking to an inconvenient bus stop or train station, and waiting there, and then having to stand

John Hillaby, the well-known English writer and naturalist, describes the pleasures to to be found in the art of walking.

for most of the journey. But even if you do not feel inspired to walk through the streets on a damp morning in December, it is a wonderful way to start a day's work when the trees are misty-green and gardens are bursting with apple blossom and forsythia.

People look happier when they are moving, purposively, on their feet. The walk to work, or an exploration of your own neighbourhood in the quiet of a Sunday morning, is a good, enjoyable way of getting to know your area, its streets and open spaces, and also the people who live there.

Many people living in large towns or their suburbs are now rediscovering the lost art of walking. How do you start? The simple answer is that you don't. Whether you realize it or not, you've been walking for most of your life. Some people clock up enormous distances without knowing it. A waitress in a busy restaurant or a nurse in a hospital ward may easily cover eight or 10 miles in a busy day—that is at least 40 a week, 160 a month or nearly 2,000 miles a year. But that is hurried skittering in short steps, often carrying a tray or a sheaf of papers.

This kind of walking is very different from the flowing movement of a shepherd in the Yorkshire Dales gathering sheep on the high tops or, say, a farm-hand strolling down to the pub for a pint in the evenings. It may look leisurely, since country folk do not like to give the impression they are ever in a hurry. But the gait is deceptive.

When he walks a countryman leans

walking

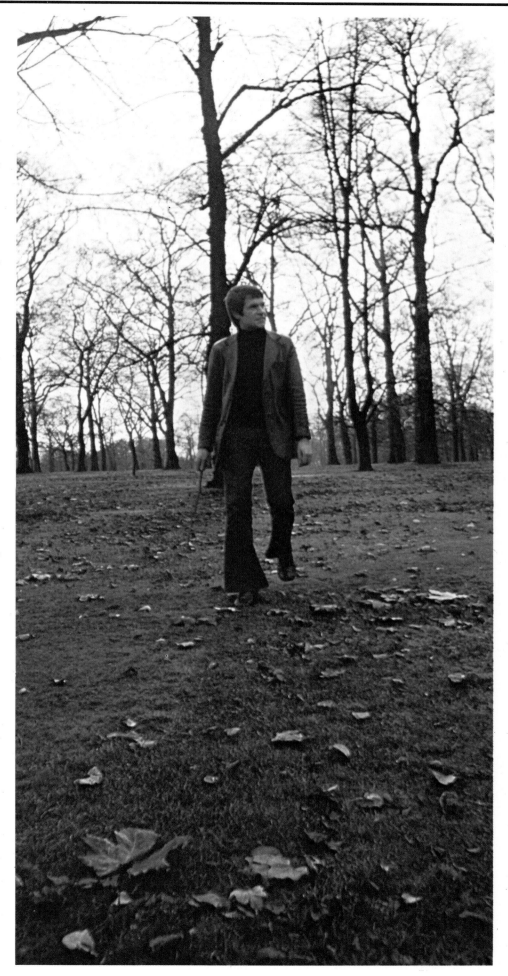

forward slightly, swinging his arms, taking relatively long strides on feet that almost brush the ground, but not quite, except maybe for the blade tips of the grass. He is in touch with his environment.

And here, I think, is a vital clue to the fine art of conscious pedestrianism. As the American writer Anatole Broyard recently observed, psychologists in the last few years seem to have discovered, as if for the first time, the importance of people touching one another, of establishing physical contact in an increasingly isolating emotional atmosphere. Touching, they suggest, is one of the few certainties still open to us. In the beginning was not the word, but the touch. In a similar spirit, sociologists and philosophers have now begun to exhort us to get back to nature, to re-integrate ourselves with our first history, and to seek the softening and soothing touch of our original mother.

A landscape is a character—and greed and affection show up more clearly on it than they do on the human face. For those of us who know what we are about, Broyard says walking "is like making love to the landscape and letting it love you back."

If that seems a high-minded or oversentimental notion of what you have been doing all your life, think about the basic dynamics of walking. Ignoring completely that gorilla-like sidewalk-scraping shuffle that some people seem to think is fashionable, imitating, perhaps, a movie gangster, the first kind of walk is the skitter or turkey trot. It is unavoidable for chores around the house, the office or the factory. It is universal. It is how the skin-clad mate of Neanderthal Man moved from one side of the cave to the other. But when her hairy partner went out hunting, perhaps following a herd of reindeer or wild horses for days and days, he would adopt a very different style of walking which is a marvel of balance, an example of what an engineer would call controlled feed-back.

At each forward step the upright human frame teeters on the edge of catastrophe. The thrust comes from the ball of the foot. But if we had to rely wholly on shoving backwards against the ground we should soon get very tired. What enables a human being to outwalk a horse is his ability to co-ordinate his gait with gravity, the fact that all small forces are attracted towards larger ones—the moon to the earth, the earth and the other planets to the sun and the sun to an almost incomprehensible profusion of super-stars. In walking we are a part of something universal.

Try this simple exercise some time. Put on a really comfortable pair of shoes. Choose a well-defined path of no less than two or three miles in length through open country so that there is no need to pick your way around obstacles or to look down too much. With your heels almost together, stand bolt upright with shoulders back but arms held limply. Lean forward until you have all but lost your balance and at that point push your right foot forward a shade further than in a normal stride and, at the same time, push back hard on the ball of your left foot. Walk on your toes for the first 10 paces, swinging your arms rhythmically. Glance down just once to ensure that your arms, with fingers slightly curled and pointing backwards, are describing an arc of about 90 degrees. If you are a wholly normal person unused to this super-charged way of walking, you'll hesitate or wobble a bit for maybe 20 or 30 paces, perhaps through self-consciousness. But walk proud—like a ballet dancer, or a Shakespearian actor in the role of a great king coming in from the wings to take his final bow.

Good walking is not only a sensuous and aesthetic exercise, but a very healthy one. In one hour, say a little under four miles, you can get more invigoration than from the same amount of time spent in a sauna bath, or on a rowing machine. And, once you have worked out your own most comfortable speed with a bit of practice, you will move easily through the gears of walking like a racing driver who reacts automatically to get the best out of his finely-tuned engine.

These gears are important. First there is what I call "ambulatory neutral." Let's assume that you are ready to set off on a fairly long cross-country walk. You have planned it. You have looked carefully at the maps or you may be accompanied by someone who knows precisely what he is about. Don't gallop off at the start. Slip into ambulatory neutral. This is the time for trimming, for adjusting rucksack straps if you are carrying a load. Fit it high with the heavy stuff on top. The pack should feel like a part of your body.

At no point from neck to toe should you be conscious of the slightest friction or discomfort. If you have a slight pinched-up feeling under your shoe-laces, for instance, you have probably tied them too tightly. Stop and loosen them. Maybe there is a slight prickly feeling under your left heel. It could be a rumpled stocking, or perhaps a bit of flint or grit no bigger than a pin-head. Stop and ferret it out because, through constant abrasion, a minute piece of grit will soon provoke a pea-sized blister which, by nightfall, will grow to the size of an overcoat button.

After a mile or two you should be in second gear—that is, at normal cruising speed. But beyond this point and infinitely superior to it, the practiced walker finds that on good days he slips almost imperceptibly into a supercharged form

of motion. He can tackle hills or walk faster with the confidence of the driver of a powerful car who knows that by a mere touch on the accelerator he can pass almost anything on the road. This does not mean that the walker necessarily increases speed. What counts is the consciousness of being able to do so without effort.

You may or may not want to storm the length of the Western Highlands of Scotland or cross the Alps on foot, although I can say from experience that this is not nearly as difficult as it sounds. But fairly soon you could be ready for something better than seven or eight miles and what applies to a marathon trek holds equally good for the South Downs Way in Sussex or anywhere where the going is wide-open and wind-swept—and

Walking can be a source of inspiration. There is something about the spring of the ground that will set your mind in motion.

always a delight, even in a light spatter of rain.

There is first and foremost the question of equipment, especially footwear. Don't be put off by all the nonsense talked about "stout boots," especially if "stout" means "heavy." Some people like them. Or need them. Or feel that dressing-up is part of the exercise—like buying a Norwegian multi-coloured sweater for a skiing trip, or a stick the weight and size of a medieval club for a walking tour.

Keep experimenting. Wear what you feel comfortable in. Make sure your footfootwear has good Commando-type or nailed treads and is waterproof. Put a wax or oil-based polish on them, both inside and out, especially under the tongue. Do not use dubbing that rots stitching. Ask your local dealer if he has got any *Veldtschoen* types of shoes or boots. These are expensive and a bit heavy, but they are the best. The uppers are doubled and in that way seal the welt, making it waterproof. Make sure they are both as strong and as light as possible.

Another simple but extremely important tip is that if you are intent on a week or a fortnight's walking, you should try to wear your shoes or boots as much as you can, if possible, all day, for at least a week before you start. Nobody will notice them under trousers.

For top clothing, choose light, windproof zipped jackets and T-shirts. Start off zipped up to your chin. As you begin to generate your own heat, unzip, gradually. Remember that over-heating is far more tiring and, in certain circumstances, almost as dangerous as being wet and cold. Don't sweat. Adjust your clothing and be comfortable the whole time. For warmth wear one or two super-light, open-weave woollen pullovers—the kind that mountaineers carry. But take them

off and stow them away as soon as you feel warm.

Rain can be a problem. There is no material known to me which is both rainproof and comfortable to walk in. If your body can breathe through it, it will not be rain-proof for long. Pack a light plastic raincoat, the bigger and airier the better. And take it off as soon as you can.

The dangers of walking out into the wilds are neither to be ignored nor exaggerated. Fatalities are relatively few, and in almost every instance, especially among parties of youngsters, these can be attributed to downright ignorance of fundamentals. Usually, the unfortunates were badly clothed. They were not carrying maps and compasses and, worst of all, they did not stop and doss down when conditions deteriorated.

The breath of the arch-killer of the unprepared is a grey-white four-letter word. It is mist. You can avoid exposure to the elements by buying a one-man tent that weighs less than two pounds. But the inexperienced should never travel alone over the highlands or moorlands. For a group of two, three or more walkers, a biggish, cheap tent can be lightly and conveniently broken down into its component parts among the party, providing, of course, that the members vow to keep together.

Why walk? There was a time—more than a thousand years ago—when Britain and the rest of Europe were criss-crossed with intercontinental trails. Whole armies marched back and forth across the Alps. Alcuin, the scholar of York, thought nothing of setting off at least once a year to have a chat with his imperial patron, Charlemagne, in Aix-la-Chapelle and then ambling down to Rome for a session with the Pope. Priestly scholars, like Clement and Durcuil, regularly trudged to Paris and Padua. St. Willibrord, the "athlete of God" from Northumbria, walked around Europe several times.

But gradually the walkers' roads became pack-horse trails and today even the great passes like the St. Gotthard and the Mont Cenis are super-highways. And yet, long before they were defiled by ferro-concrete and petrol fumes, men thought it worth their while to keep to their feet. Victorian sermons were composed in the vicarage walk. The lake poets were inspired on the top of the fells. There is something about the spring of the ground that sets your mind in motion.

Where can you walk? You can still walk almost anywhere, if you know how to set about it. In England the Pennine Way, the Ridgeway in Wessex, the North and South Downs and innumerable coastal paths are reasonably well blazed and sign-posted. There are networks of trails in the United States and numerous *sentiers* in western Europe. All over the world there are walking clubs which can guide you to high adventure. Get out on your feet! Even if you just resolve to walk to work for a change, you can discover a new dimension in life.

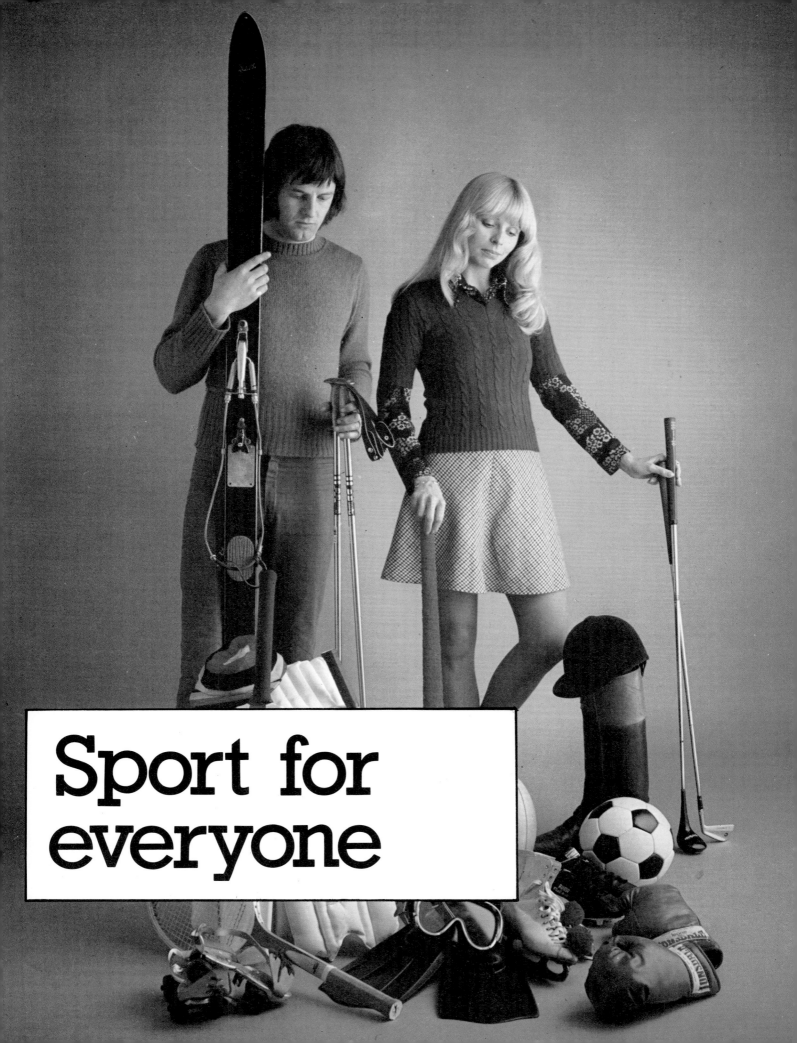

Sport for everyone

Sport and recreation

Sir Winston Churchill avoided physical exertion whenever it was possible. And he lived to be 91 years old. Lesser mortals, however, are unlikely to be endowed with longevity if they follow his example.

The Framingham Study, conducted in a small town in Massachusetts, has shown that the incidence of coronary thrombosis in those people who have little or no recreational exercise is substantially higher than the rate among those who exercise regularly.

Exercise is a natural need of the human body. That stretching yawn first thing in the morning, itself a form of exercise, is demonstrating an unconscious need to stretch the muscles and put the body to work. It is followed by a slight relaxation, a give of the muscle tissues. However reluctantly acknowledged, the body is expressing a desire for activity. And, for most of us, that desire is rarely satisfied.

Exercise, in any form, improves balance and co-ordination and helps to keep the muscles in trim. A gradual increase in the amount of exertion will improve strength, stamina and endurance. Those forms of exercise which demand a wide range of movement increase the mobility of the joints. The vigorous breathing and acceleration of the pulse rate that results from exercise promotes the efficiency of the heart and increases the capacity of the lungs.

Any exercise steps up the respiratory rate and promotes deeper breathing. A greater quantity of oxygen is taken in and passed into the bloodstream with a revitalizing effect. On exhalation, unwelcome amounts of carbon dioxide are discharged.

Most people who have been persuaded to participate in some kind of strenuous exercise are surprised when they discover that afterwards they feel invigorated and less tired than they did before they began. This feeling of restored vitality is one of the best arguments for involvement in meaningful physical activity.

With a reserve, a credit balance of energy, strength and skill, it is easier to make further worthwhile and enjoyable activities part of our total programme of living. Maintaining the flexibility of both mind and body requires practice. But just as intellectual stimulation is necessary for the mind, so physical exertion is a necessity for the body.

But what kind of exercise, and how much, is right for you? It is a complex task to determine this because it depends on so many factors, including your physique, sex, age, occupation, natural skills and personal preferences.

Perhaps the most basic and over-riding criteria is your body type. A look at the runners in an Olympic marathon would immediately convince most large and overweight people that that form of exercise was not for them. And a thin, light person would not fare too well in a rowing crew.

The broad classification of body types made by William Sheldon in the United States in 1940 can help to determine the range of activities most suitable to the individual.

Mesomorphs, those with well-built, athletic bodies, have the widest choice. Nearly the whole range of sports, games and outdoor activities is open to them. These strong, muscular people are restricted only by the factors which may affect everyone—lack of ability, money or facilities, and their own preferences.

Ectomorphs, those with slender physiques, are obviously limited to areas of exercise where strength or bulk are unimportant. But they frequently excel in those activities which require either stamina, skill or intense concentration. Ectomorphs have been described as keenly aware of their environment and not very socially inclined. They might,

---

Heart attacks are twice as common among office workers as they are among manual workers. Although both need exercise, it is clear who needs most. But how much, and what kind?

---

therefore, be best suited to such individual specialist sports as long-distance running or mountaineering.

Endomorphs, those with soft, well-rounded bodies and a marked tendency to be overweight, are also limited in their choice. Such activities as bowling and golf (which also make use of the endomorph's natural gregariousness) are probably preferable to strenuous exercise and the rigours of fierce competition.

Another major factor in the choice and amount of exercise is occupation. There is clearly a great difference between the exercise requirements of a person whose work involves physical exertion and one whose job confines him to a desk for most of the day. A study of American railwaymen revealed that the rate of coronary thrombosis, for example, was considerably higher among the clerks than it was among the platelayers.

Normally the office worker will not get sufficient exercise during his five day week. The average male office worker expends about 2,600 calories a day, compared with the 3,700 of the coal miner. Because he spends most of his time sitting, he may develop postural faults—a flat chest, round shoulders, round back and the weak abdominal muscles which lead to paunchiness. The buttock and thigh muscles of a sedentary worker may also suffer from lack of use. Vigorous and frequent exercise in his

leisure time is necessary to compensate for the disabilities caused by his work.

The manual worker, on the other hand, will generally be in better physical condition than his white-collar counterpart. But while his particular job may develop certain physical attributes, it may not produce a very high level of overall fitness. A road worker, for example, will develop strong arms and legs, but he may well find that if he suddenly tries any exercise involving strenuous and wide-ranging movement his particular type of fitness acquired at work is not a great help. He will be more fit than a non-exercising office worker, but new muscles and functions will come into play. He, too, needs more general exercise.

The housewife, of course, is also a worker. A woman who weighs 120 pounds and is engaged in active housework uses up about 240 calories an hour, twice the amount expended if she was playing golf or expended by a typist of the same weight. As the housewife acquires modern labour-saving equipment, however, she reduces the stretching and bending which had perhaps helped her to keep in good shape. This is not to suggest that she should give up her vacuum cleaner and electric mixer for the carpet brush and the wooden spoon; but she may need to spend some of the time she saves participating in a sport or an exercise class.

In general, women have different exercise requirements from men. A woman wants to keep her body supple and her muscles firm, to have good posture and move gracefully. Although she needs a certain degree of strength to cope with her work and daily tasks, she usually tries to avoid over-developing visible muscles, such as the thighs and upper arms, and concentrates on producing a more shapely body.

Age is another of the major factors in determining how much and what kind of exercise an individual needs. All too often, our age is given away by the way we move. Most people, as they get older, drastically reduce the amount of exercise they get and many, if they have participated in a sport, give it up. The result is a gradual stiffening of the joints and a reduction in the flexibility of the muscles.

But there is no need to abandon exercise in middle age. Indeed, there is no real foundation for the widespread belief that weight gain, or any kind of physical deterioration, is an inevitable part of growing older. That is the very time when the need for exercise to maintain the same weight and stay in condition is paramount. It is vital to exercise regularly and for as long a period of time as possible. There may be an imperceptible slowing down in the pace and intensity of the activity involved, but this in no way lessens the revitalizing effect of the exercise, nor should it lessen the enjoyment derived from it.

The other factors which may determine your possible patterns of exercise are more practical. Convenience and practicability are major influences. The nearest yachting facilities may be hours away from your home, but you may well have tennis courts or a swimming pool just around the corner. Cost, too, is often used as an excuse for not exercising. Yet, while some sports may be ruled out on the grounds of expensive equipment, travel or club fees (golf, skiing or riding perhaps), most activities cost little. And walking, the simplest form of exercise, costs nothing at all.

Almost all sports, of course, entail some sort of competitive spirit. More than one other person, and usually several, are involved. In many cases it is difficult to take up a sport or game without joining a club or society. Exercise, then, has a strong social element—sharing your experiences and enjoyment with others, both old friends and new acquaintances, and relaxing in a warm feeling of achievement and satisfaction.

This is relaxation in the most valuable sense: the opportunity to lift ourselves out of the daily routine with something completely different, the relief from the stagnating pressures and monotonous repetition of everyday life by doing something that is worthwhile, constructive and rewarding. When the problems of the daily round are faced again it is with new reserves of energy.

The sense of sharing a common goal is an important factor in becoming fit. For those who cannot or do not want to pursue the sports available to them, it is possible to join an exercise class. There the competitive element is eliminated, but the atmosphere of shared experience remains. As in slimming, where it is often easier to stay on a diet if you can compare your results with a friend, so it is more enjoyable to share your exercise programme.

Another alternative is courses which can be undertaken at home. Yoga (also very popular in classes) is the best known

The variety of sports, games, leisure activities and exercise programmes is endless. If you are unfit, it only remains for you to assess the facts and make your choice.

and now has a huge following. Its great advantage, in addition to simultaneously improving all the body's functions, is that it relaxes and refreshes the mind. Another ancient Eastern exercise system, Tai Chi, a sequence of graceful movements which exercise every part of the body by constantly shifting its balance, is rapidly winning adherents in the West.

There are, of course, numerous kinds of basic as well as more sophisticated keep-fit programmes, some done to music, some incorporating dancing, some employing exercise equipment. Isometrics, static muscular contractions using immovable objects, can also be useful, although their application is limited to the development of strength rather than general fitness. Indoor sports and games involving movement of any beneficial range are uncommon, simply because of restricted space, but table tennis can be a useful year-round activity for the whole family.

If the idea of organized physical activity, whether collective or individual, does not appeal to you, the easiest way to make sure that you get more exercise is to adopt or extend a leisure activity. Energetic gardening, for example, uses up about 2.3 calories per pound per hour, comparing favourably with 2.2 calories per pound per hour for moderate dancing or 2.1 for skating. For sawing wood, perhaps the most energetic feature of carpentry, the figure is 3.1—as much as for tennis.

With the whole range of sports, games, exercise courses and leisure activities available for every conceivable type of person and their preferences, it only remains for those people who do not get regular exercise to make their choice and then exert self-discipline and will-power to begin. Like giving up smoking, of course, it is easier said than done. But, once accomplished, the continued sense of achievement and well-being brings great satisfaction.

In attempting to establish how much exercise you need, you should keep in mind the pointlessness of the short, sharp burst of activity so often indulged in by the holiday-maker, who for a few weeks drives his flabby, under-exercised body into a state of exhaustion and then does nothing for the rest of the year. Moderate but regular activity is without doubt the most valuable and sensible approach.

It should be emphasized that, whatever your age, you must begin exercising very gradually if you are out of condition. You could do untold damage by suddenly taking up an energetic sport. The body must first be familiarized with extra movement by light exercise—walking, free-standing exercises or, perhaps, jogging.

We all need exercise. We are denying ourselves a natural desire, just like eating or sex, if we ignore this fact. How much exercise, above a certain minimum, and what kind, within individual restrictions, is up to the person concerned. For the vast majority of us there is no excuse for being anything but physically fit.

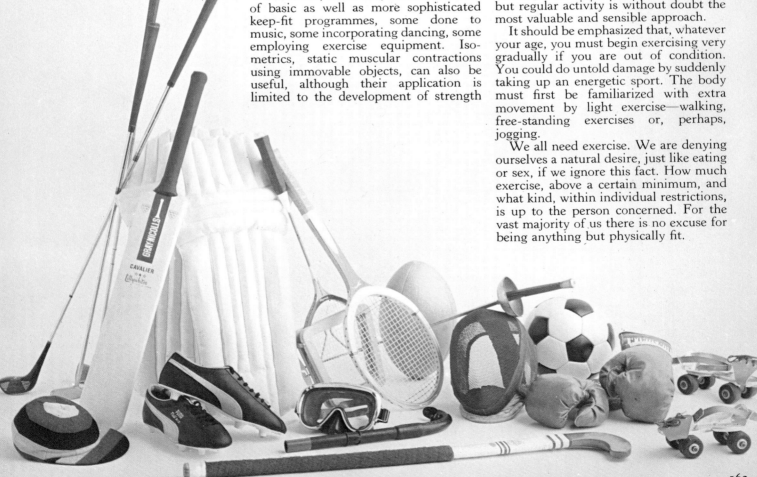

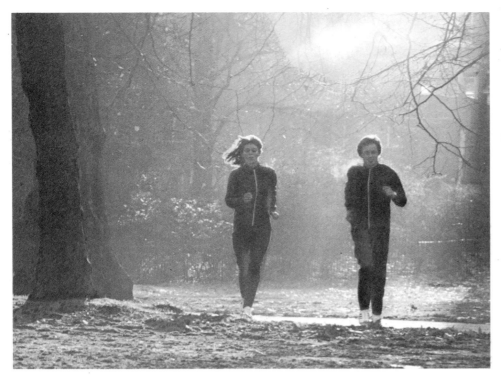

Jog for your health

Jogging is one of the most effective and simplest forms of exercise. It involves the whole body and is particularly beneficial to the heart and lungs. It requires no special skill and can be done with little inconvenience to your daily routine.

Jogging has many attractions. It can be done anywhere—in the back garden, on the beach, in the local park and even on the street. It exercises the vital bodily functions, revitalizing the heart and lungs, toning up the muscles and aiding the digestive system. Through regular jogging you can reach a peak of fitness and health which will enable you not only to perform physical tasks with greater zest but also to have a clearer mind and feel less sluggish.

The body works best when it is mobile. Tension builds up in the muscles when you are sitting or standing still. When the muscles are actually working this tension is channelled and alleviated. Jogging is one of the most natural ways to set the body in motion, to release tension in a rhythmic and vigorous way.

How does jogging exercise the heart? The heart consists of two pumps working in unison to circulate vital blood to all parts of the body. Blood returning from the body through the veins flows into the right side of the heart. From there it is pumped into the lungs where the red blood cells dispose of carbon dioxide and pick up oxygen. From the lungs, this cleansed, re-oxygenated blood returns to the left side of the heart and is then pumped to all areas of the body.

Although the heart weighs only one two-hundredth of the total body weight, it requires one-twentieth of the total blood in the body to supply it with nourishment and oxygen so that it can function at its best. The heart does not depend on the blood in its chambers for nourishment. Rather, it is continually fed by two arteries which encircle it and provide the muscles of the chambers with oxygen-laden blood.

The power needed to pump from the heart is supplied by the myocardium, a muscle system surrounding the chambers of the heart. When the myocardium relaxes blood is pumped into the heart, when it contracts the blood is forced out. The efficiency of the heart is very dependent on the ability of the myocardium to relax and contract with added capacity.

Jogging increases the capacity of the myocardium, enabling it to work with greater force so that the heart relaxes more completely and contracts with more strength, emptying and filling the chambers more thoroughly. When the heart is working to its full capacity, the myocardium pumps more blood. This increase in the beat volume enables the heart to pump more blood while beating at a much slower rate. The rest period between beats becomes longer and more beneficial.

Jogging is one of the most effective ways of exercising the myocardium and improving the whole circulatory system. By following a jogging programme you can actually increase the size and power of this very important muscle and ensure,

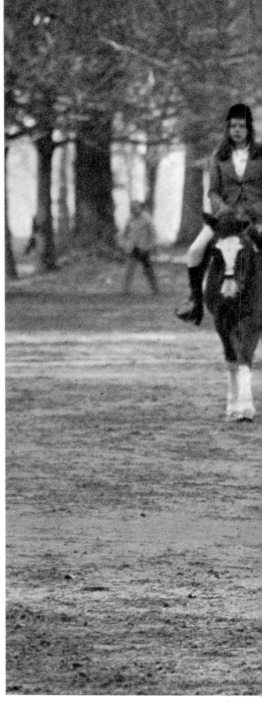

barring the misfortune of ill-health, that you will be free of most forms of heart disease which attack middle-aged people. Even if you are young this kind of exercise could very well be vital at a later stage in your life.

Heart disease is the largest single cause of death. To a large extent, the premature degeneration of the heart can be attributed to the sedentary, non-athletic lives which most of us lead. By not making demands on our muscles we set in train certain degenerative processes.

The first sign of such deterioration is usually obesity. Fat is the energy supply of the body. If it is not used it is stored.

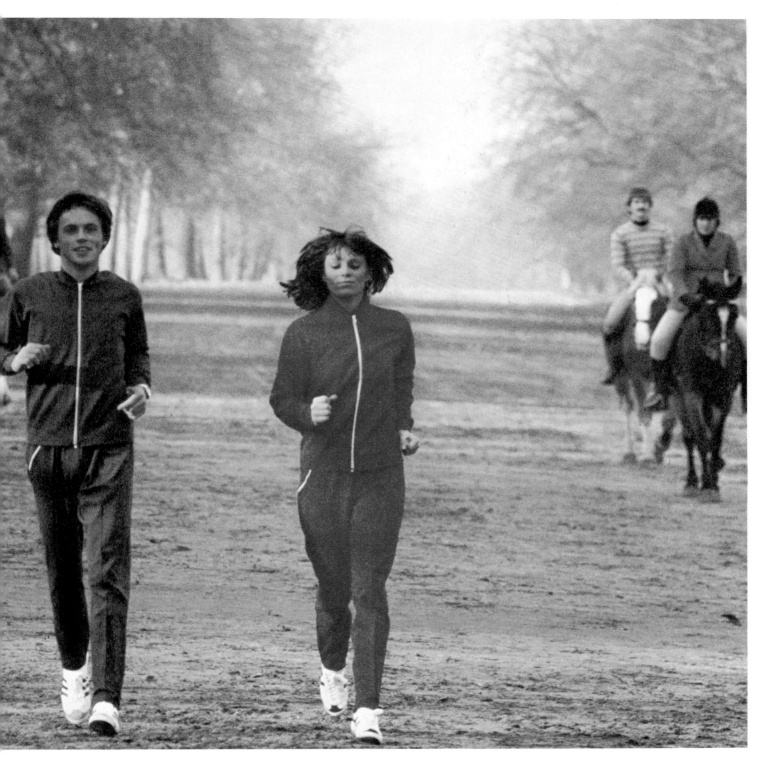

Although eating habits have a great deal to do with overweight problems, exercise is also an important factor. Exercise consumes a good proportion of fat. This is because exercise forces the lungs into working at something near their true capacity. While you are sitting or standing, your lungs are only being used at about a quarter of their potential. If the other three-quarters are continuously unused they will cease to maintain their vital capacity. When more oxygen is needed by the heart and other muscles in the body, the lungs will need to work extra hard in their reduced state.

The muscles of your body need oxygen in order to convert fat into energy. If the muscles do not make demands on the heart and lungs, these will atrophy—that is, they will become weaker and have a reduced capacity. The circulatory system is also affected. If there is not at least an occasional demand for extra oxygen from hard-working muscles and a corresponding increase in the rate and volume of blood flowing through arteries, capillaries and veins to supply it, all of these blood vessels begin to narrow in diameter. The circulatory system with its smaller channels and sluggish blood flow can then become clogged with fats and cholesterol. (Cholesterol is a poten-

tially deadly fatty substance). The arteries in the heart are not immune from this degeneration. It is when fats and cholesterol begin to clog the heart itself that the greatest danger arises. A heart attack and even possible death may ensue.

Jogging uses most muscles in the body, especially those in the legs. The lungs are forced to breathe in more oxygen to feed the muscles; the heart has to beat faster to supply this oxygen to the muscles. In this way the whole circulatory system is cleansed and brought to a higher peak of capacity.

It has been shown that regular exercise increases the diameter of the capillaries

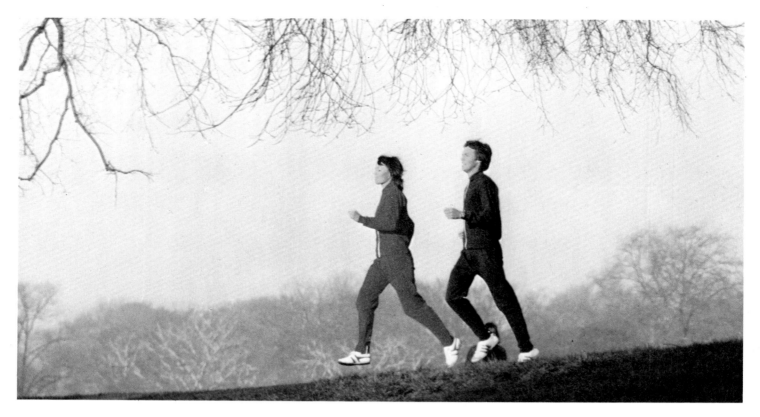

by 100 per cent and the number of capillaries by 400 per cent. To improve your level of fitness and reach a renewed state of health you must increase your pulse rate to between 120 and 140 beats per minute for at least 15 minutes each day. Jogging is one of the most effective ways of doing this.

Jogging is also an extremely enjoyable way of releasing mental tension. The physical rhythm, the controlled breathing and the repetition perform the same function as simple meditation exercises. The extra oxygen in the body goes to the brain as well as to the active leg muscles. After you have tried jogging you will notice a new ease of mind and will be better able to cope with stress.

Jogging is a physical experience which gives the mind something wholesome and uncomplicated to concentrate on. Because of this it will enable you to be mentally and physically fit. Lack of fitness is a conscious as well as an unconscious source of anxiety. By achieving a high level of fitness you can refresh your whole attitude to life. Your metabolism is improved. You eat less. You lead a more active life.

One of the main attractions of jogging is that it can be done anywhere and at any time. You will probably find that early in the morning before a shower and breakfast is a good time to go jogging. In the evening after work is also a convenient time. The beneficial effects of an evening jog are really appreciated. The cares and stresses which have accumulated over the course of the day will disappear as if by magic.

How should you begin a jogging programme? Start by combining jogging with walking for periods of 15 minutes.

JOGGING FOR WOMEN

Jogging is usually thought of as a predominantly male form of exercise. There is no reason, however, that women should not become involved. It is an excellent means of removing excessive weight and keeping your body in shapely trim. Start with the following jogging session.

Carry out some light exercises. Then break into a slow trot for a quarter of a mile. Continue for another quarter of a mile in a steady jog. When you begin to feel tired, walk for about 100 yards. When you have recovered your breath start to trot again for another quarter of a mile. Gradually increase your speed to a steady jog. Continue this for half a mile. When you find this too demanding, slow down into a trot and finally begin to walk for 100 yards.

You should not find this programme too difficult. If you do, reduce the distances by a half. If you think that you are not expending enough effort, double the distances.

Do not over-exert yourself at first. As you become fitter you will be able to redouble your efforts without undue strain. If you feel too much at ease, however, you will not gain the full benefits of jogging.

Over a period of time, gradually reduce the amount of walking you find necessary until you eliminate it completely. Then increase the exercise time to half an hour, again combining walking with jogging. Slowly cut down on the walking time. The time you devote to jogging, however, is completely up to your own individual needs and likes.

Jogging is free and easy. There are no set rules. The distance you cover, the time you spend and the ease with which you jog are entirely guided by your ability and capacity. A good rule of thumb is to judge the speed and distance of your jog by how your heart and whole body reacts. You should feel that you are making an effort. But as soon as you begin to notice that your heart is beating very quickly and that you feel uncomfortable, start to walk. If you feel that jogging might cause you to over-strain your heart because of a previous illness, it is advisable to seek the advice of a doctor before starting.

As your fitness improves you will feel the need to exert yourself a little more. So either increase your distance by jogging a little faster or allow yourself more time. The important thing to remember is that you should progress gradually, never putting unnecessary stress on the heart.

How often you should jog also depends on your personal preferences, time and ability. Many physical fitness experts believe that you should jog every day. But there is no reason to follow this if you do not have the time or if you feel that such a programme would over-exert your body. If you feel this is the case why not jog on alternate days? This allows for a 'recovery' day in between. Perhaps the best programme to follow is to jog just when you feel like it.

It is a good idea to combine your jogging with some form of light exercise programme. You could, for example, do some calisthenics before going out to jog. Or, if you liked, devote some time to hatha yoga postures when you have returned from your jogging session. Exercises after jogging are necessary because of factors affecting the circulation.

Blood being pumped out of the heart is assisted in its flow by the muscular contractions of the arteries. After the blood has flowed through the capillaries at the end of the arteries, however, it goes into the veins to return to the heart. Unlike arteries, the veins do not have any muscles in their walls to keep the blood continually flowing along. They have a series of one-way valves which keep the blood flowing only towards the heart. Movement is necessary to keep the blood in the veins flowing towards the heart. This is because every time you move a muscle it contracts the nearest veins and causes the blood to flow in the direction of the heart.

Lack of muscle movement in the legs means that blood almost remains station-

JOGGING FOR MEN

After doing a small amount of preliminary exercises, begin your jog with a quarter mile trot.
Then break into a jogging rhythm for about half a mile. When you begin to feel tired or ill at ease it is advisable to spend a period of time just walking. This will allow you to catch your breath.
When you have recovered your breath, begin to jog again for another half mile. Maintain an even steady pace.
Walk for about 100 yards to regain your breath.
This is an easy-to-follow jogging session. It should make no excessive demands on your stamina and endurance.
For a harder jog, double the distances given above. Do not attempt any great distances at first. Wait until you have been jogging for some time.

ary in the legs and abdomen. This is the reason why some form of exercise is necessary after you have jogged. While you are jogging a great amount of blood is sent to the legs. Therefore a period of light exercise will help to redistribute this blood through the whole body. These exercises should last for at least five minutes.

The form which these exercises should take is entirely up to you. They do not have to be any specific set of exercises. The important thing is that you move the top part of the body as much as possible after your jogging session.

Jogging brings many benefits, pleasures and satisfaction both to men and women. For the little amount of effort and thought you have to put into it you will gain an over-abundance of health and well-being, both of body and of mind. Resolve to start a jogging programme now. Remember that all you need to jog is the decision to start.

The time you devote to jogging, whether it is great or small, will bring you plenty of enjoyment as well as a refreshing release from the tensions which affect your mind and body. Remember as with all exercise, take it slowly at first.

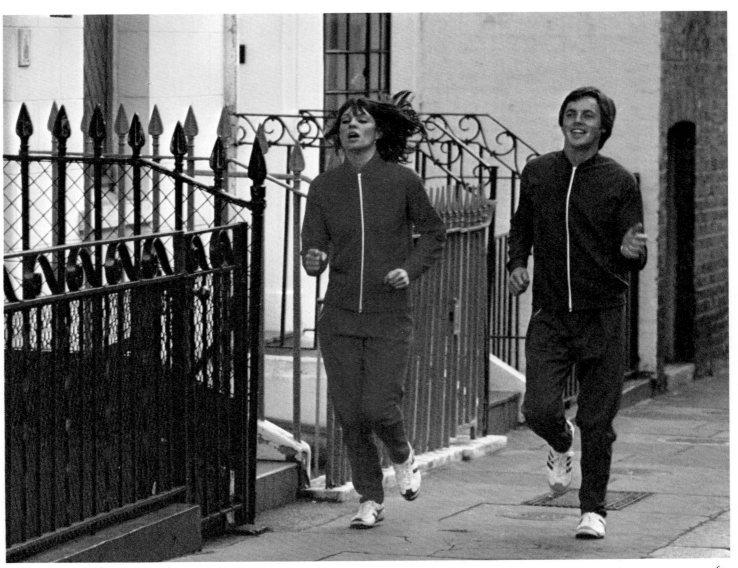

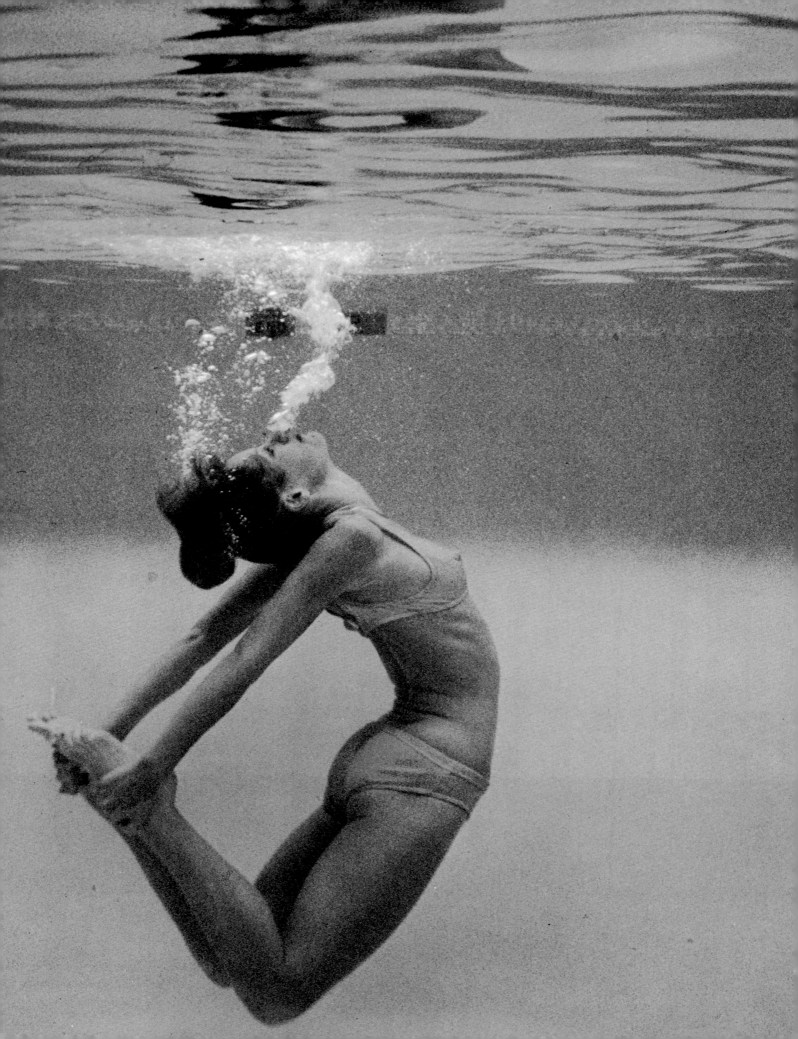

Swimming—The Total Exercise

There is probably no other single activity which is more pleasurable or more beneficial than swimming. As a general exercise it promotes the action of almost every muscle in the body, stimulates circulation of the blood and improves the efficiency of the heart and lungs. And swimming is easy to learn, accessible and inexpensive.

As a useful skill swimming is applicable to innumerable human situations. Nobody, anywhere in the world, is far from some body of water and although the necessity of being a capable swimmer is obvious for people who live near the sea, lakes, rivers or canals, there does come a time in almost everyone's life when the confident ability to swim is invaluable—even to the point of saving a life.

Besides the safety factor, swimming has many other advantages. It would be difficult, for example, to fully enjoy a seaside holiday without being able to swim. And it is almost impossible to join a sailing or rowing club without first proving that you can swim well. There are many exciting activities, too, for which the ability to swim is a prerequisite. These include scuba diving, sub-aqua swimming, surfing, synchronized swimming (a form of water ballet) and water-polo.

Another advantage of swimming is that it is an individual skill and can be enjoyed alone. And age is no barrier. People of any age and in almost every state of health can learn to swim. For the disabled and physically handicapped swimming is an ideal exercise. The buoyant nature of the human body makes it possible for even the severely disabled to achieve a mobility in water that they lack on land. Physical strength is not necessary, but swimming does promote muscle elasticity and strength.

People who are overweight also benefit from swimming and they swim easily since fat is light. Because long ranging movement of the muscles is involved, swimming, as part of a weight-reduction programme which includes a sensible diet, is ideally suited to women who want to lose weight.

Most people are familiar with the four strokes used in competitive swimming— breaststroke, backstroke, butterfly and the front crawl or freestyle. The breaststroke is the oldest recorded swimming stroke and in fact Aristotle recommended that those wishing to learn to swim study the motion of frogs. Oddly he was wrong, for the human breaststroke is fundamentally different from the frog's movements. The arms and legs propel the body forward alternately, and the arms pull while the legs prepare to kick backwards; the legs push backwards with the inside of the foot while the arms stretch forward ready to pull. The body is flat on the water and the face and mouth need never be put underwater.

Although at competition level the breaststroke is demanding, it is ideal for recreational swimming. A good speed can be built up by using the legs to propel and the arms merely to stabilize and help in breathing—the breaststroke is the only one of the four competitive strokes in which the legs are as useful as the arms— and speed can be increased if the arms are used more strenuously.

The breaststroke is the basic technique used in life-saving and in personal

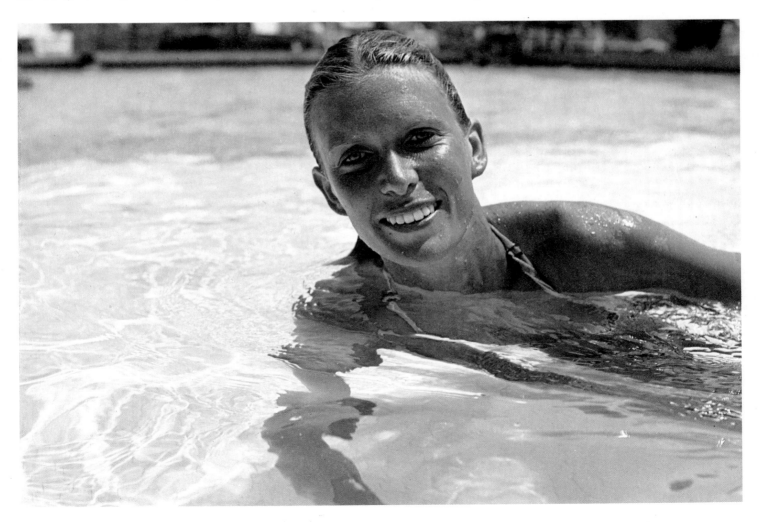

survival. Its advantages are that it relies heavily on the legs—and most people's legs are stronger and have more endurance than their arms—and that the arms never come above the surface of the water. (When the arms and legs come above the surface they become heavier and more difficult and tiring to move.)

The butterfly is really a development of the breaststroke. In the 1920's and 1930's frustrated and competitive breast-stroke swimmers took advantage of a legal loophole and began their arm recovery (the non-propelling phase of a stroke) over the water. This was so much faster than the orthodox breaststroke that the new stroke was legalized and the rules of the breaststroke were tightened up to save it from oblivion. The butterfly is, however, essentially a competitive technique and it is strenuous and difficult. But if you can master it you will improve your general ability in the water.

The butterfly is, like the breaststroke, swum on the front. The arms recover over the surface of the water, and pull strongly under the body to pull the body forward and to lift the mouth above the water for breathing. The legs perform an up-and-down dolphin movement which balances the body, compensates for the strong pull of the arms, and helps the head to lift in order to breathe.

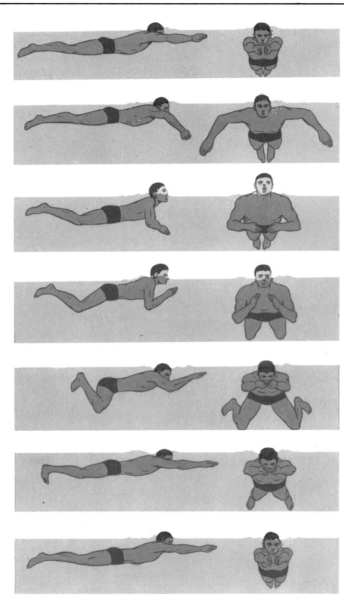

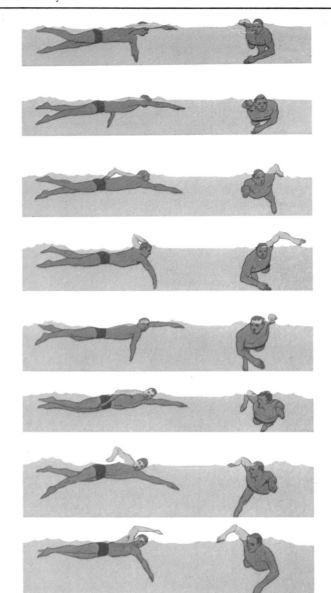

BREASTSTROKE

In the breaststroke the body is kept as flat as possible, with the head lifting above the water only to inhale. The arms pull while the legs "recover," as the non-propelling part of a stroke is known, and the arms recover close to the chest to cut down resistance. The drive in the legs, made as the arms push forward, comes from the downward kick of the shins, the rotational kick of the instep and the backward thrust of the feet.

FRONT CRAWL

The freestyle, or more accurately the front crawl, is the fastest of the swimming strokes, but the legs use only a shallow flutter kick which gives more stability than propulsion. On entry into the water the hand sinks a few inches to the 'catch point', where the arm starts its propelling action. The swimmer then pulls and pushes himself past the hand, which tends to remain stationary. The recovery of the arm over the water allows a period of relaxation, while the swimmer breathes with the head to one side. It is important to keep the body flat, with the buttocks well up.

The earliest competitive backstroke was known as the Old English backstroke, a kind of inverted breaststroke in which the legs did the same backward double thrust and the arms pulled sideways down past the body and recovered over the water to a position above the head. This was superseded by the modern backcrawl stroke in which the arms pull alternately in a windmill fashion and the legs move alternately.

The back crawl is an ideal introduction to the front crawl stroke because the legs kick in the same manner and the alternating rhythm of the stroke is similar. But in this stroke, unlike the breaststroke, the arms do most of the propelling while the legs balance the body. Some people prefer the backstroke to others because the face and mouth are always above the surface of the water and breathing requires no special effort.

The fastest swimming technique is the front crawl stroke. The arms pull alternately under the body and can move more powerfully than in the lateral movements of the backstroke. The legs simply balance and stabilize, although they do provide some motion.

Most people, when they are learning the front crawl, find the breathing a bit difficult. They have an instinctive desire to lift their heads upwards and, in the

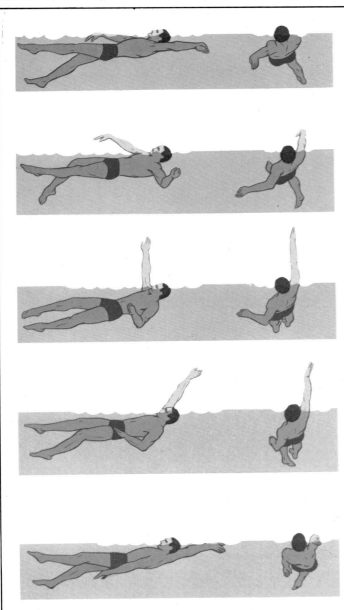

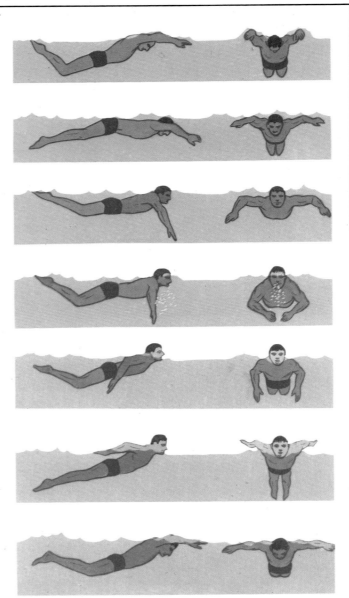

BACKSTROKE

The arm action is vitally important in the backstroke, with the hand following the shape of a lengthened 'S'. The pull starts as the arm enters the water and 'catches hold' of the water about six inches below the surface. The hand pulls back and, as the arm bends, the forearm rotates. The recovery of the arm is a relaxed and smooth movement. The head and body should be kept flat. The legs normally kick six times to one cycle of the arms, and should not go deeper into the water than 18 inches or two feet.

BUTTERFLY

A flowing rhythm is necessary for a good butterfly stroke. The arms provide most of the power, but they cannot work effectively without the stabilizing action of the legs and body. There are two distinct dolphin leg movements — a large beat before the arms recover, which provides some propulsion, and a balancing beat as the arms pass the shoulders. The arms pull diagonally outwards and then in towards the stomach. They then slip sideways and are lifted low over the water. Breathing occurs when the head is lifted. When inhalation is complete the head is dropped to ease the recovery.

front crawl, the breath is taken to the side.

Apart from the four competitive strokes there are others which are easy to learn and fun to do. The Old English backstroke is one example. Another, which is suited to long, relaxed swims, is the sidestroke.

If you try to swim breaststroke on your side and succeed, the chances are that you will be swimming sidestroke. The legs kick with a strong scissor movement and if you are on your left side the right arm recovers over the water and the left arm underwater. In the sidestroke, the face is always clear of the water, and it's a good stroke in choppy water where the front crawl is often ineffective and the breaststroke is too slow.

Each of these swimming strokes has its application and advantages. The speed of the front crawl, for example, cannot be surpassed by any other stroke; the breaststroke and the sidestroke are excellent for ease of movement and endurance. The backstroke provides a pleasant change from the front crawl. Mastery of the Old English backstroke is essential in life-saving. Only the butterfly stroke is not very useful for the non-competitor.

Swimming is a total exercise and swimming regularly will make you healthier and more physically fit.

One of the great advantages of swimming is that it employs almost every muscle in the body. In the front crawl and the butterfly the same muscles are used. These include those of the upper and lower arms, the shoulder muscles and those in the upper chest, abdomen and back. The leg actions greatly exercise the muscles in the buttocks and the front of the thighs.

In the breaststroke the leg muscles are exercised more than they are in the front crawl. This stroke is also particularly recommended for people who have back trouble because of its gentle exercising of the back muscles.

The arm pull in the backstroke utilizes the same muscles as the front crawl, but in a different direction and with a different emphasis.

The muscles of the neck play an important role in all the strokes. The head must be turned, for example, in the front crawl, lifted in the breaststroke and the butterfly, and kept still in the backstroke and sidestroke.

Doctors and physiotherapists are always quick to point out that the same movements required to swim, if done out of water, are neither as effective nor as beneficial and require greater effort than they do in water.

Swimming is an easy and pleasant way to exercise and there is no reason why any normally fit person should not enjoy it. It can be learned easily, at any age, and once learned is never forgotten. But merely mastering the basic strokes will not enable you to control your body in heavy surf or to swim steadily for a long period of time. That requires practice.

Assuming you are healthy you can work out a swimming programme over a period of six months or a year which will make you more than just a competent swimmer, give you the benefit of total physical exercise and improve your general fitness. (Anyone, however, who suffers from asthma, cardiac trouble, or has any other physical complaint should discuss the advisability of a swimming programme with his or her doctor.)

It is best to find a pool where you can swim regularly. It does not take very much time and you can set aside several lunch hours each week or plan to swim early in the mornings or in the evenings. All that is required is that you can do, and not necessarily very well, the three basic strokes—the front crawl, the breaststroke and the backstroke. Even two strokes will do—the breaststroke and the backstroke.

It will take several sessions before you become accustomed to moving easily in the water and discover all those muscles you didn't know you had. Begin by swimming 30 minutes a session, and set

SAFETY AND SWIMMING

To fully enjoy swimming you should know and follow the simple rules of safety in the water.
1 Avoid swimming alone. The best swimmers can get into difficulties.
2 Never swim in areas where you are advised not to. Only swim in the sea if that part of the coast is considered safe.
3 Try to stay in your depth if you're not confident.
4 Never swim if there is a strong under-tow.
5 If you are caught in a current, don't swim against it. Swim obliquely across it. It will be easier to walk back than to swim.
6 Don't swim out to sea. Remember, it's easier to get out than to get back.
7 Don't swim outdoors for too long, especially if it is cold. This particularly applies to the sea.
8 Don't swim immediately after you have eaten. A stomach cramp, particularly in the sea, is extremely dangerous.
9 Don't panic if you're in trouble. Don't waste your energy shouting and waving. If you have a cramp, stretch the muscle.
10 Never swim after drinking alcohol. Rather than keep you warm, it promotes the flow of blood to your skin, leaving your internal organs short of blood and prone to cold.

as your first goal a continuous swim of 200 metres. Then work up to 200 metres doing a front stroke and 200 metres doing a back stroke.

If you swim two or three times a week you should soon work up to that level. Once you have achieved this, begin to measure how fast you can swim. Most swimming pools have a clock with a second hand which is used by swimmers who are training for competition. Use that to time yourself, or ask someone to time you, over any distance up to 100 metres, which should take you about two minutes. Remember the time and, every week or so, try it again. You will be surprised how quickly you will improve your time.

You should soon be capable of swimming up to 800 metres, or half a mile, without a break. You can vary your training (for that is what you're doing) by concentrating on a different stroke each session and by learning new skills, such as swimming the butterfly, swimming underwater (where the breaststroke is recommended), and practising racing turns.

After a few months of regular practice you should improve your time for 100 metres by about 20 seconds. And if you can beat 100 seconds for 100 metres breaststroke you are doing very well. The front crawl and the backstroke are usually faster strokes. About 85 seconds for 100 metres on these strokes is very good.

You will probably, at some point, reach a plateau. But don't be discouraged if you don't improve for several weeks: this is common to many sports and not peculiar to swimming. When this happens go on to a different stroke and work on it or try swimming a medley—one stroke for one length of the pool, another stroke back and so on.

After six months of a regular swimming programme you will be a good swimmer. You can then concentrate on maintaining a satisfactory level of performance and continue to swim regularly to ensure that you keep the level of physical fitness you have achieved.

Every competent swimmer should also take a course in life-saving, which teaches the techniques and subtleties of rescuing and reviving a drowning person or someone who has got into difficulties in the water. Many new aspects of swimming, including scuba diving, will also be opened up to you. There are adult education classes which give courses both in life-saving and other swimming-orientated activities.

There is also the encouraging and true story of the man, not a very good swimmer, whose friends bet him that he couldn't swim the English Channel—well over 20 miles. They lost their money.

Anybody can swim and everybody should swim. And it's never too late to learn. Regular swimming is beneficial to your health. It will keep you physically fit and best of all, swimming is fun and can be enjoyed by people of all ages.

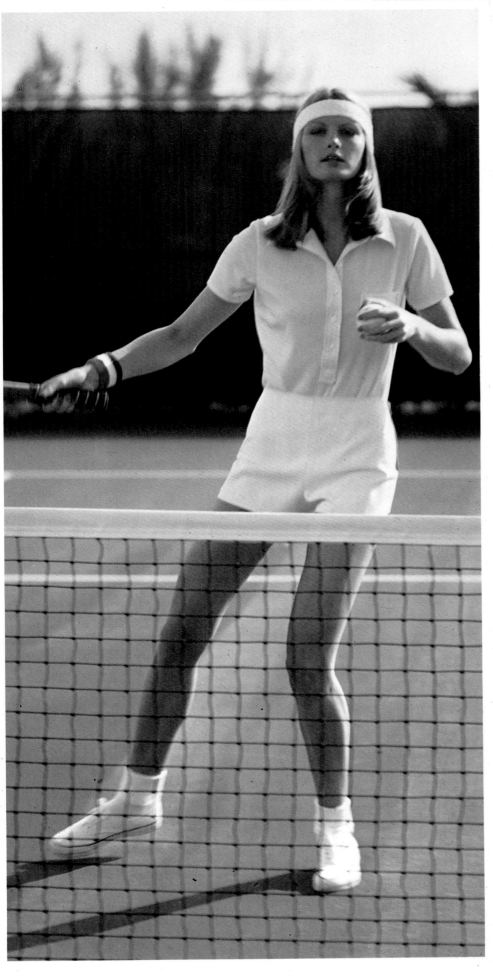

Sports & Games You can Enjoy

Taking part in sports and games is one of the most enjoyable ways of keeping fit—and of meeting people. Whether it's going to the park for a game of tennis with a friend, joining a team or a club and playing regularly, or spending a day sailing or riding, sports and games extend the benefits of on-the-spot exercises and have many other advantages.

There is a wide variety of sports and games. Take part in one you enjoy—it will provide good exercise and continued entertainment.

A sport is often more enjoyable than an exercise routine just because it involves other people. You see old friends and meet new ones while keeping fit. Competition can help, too. The result may be unimportant, but the incentive to be that little better can make exertion easier. And the interest of the activity itself draws from your efforts which develop your skills, improve your balance and co-ordination, increase your poise and suppleness, and leave you fitter—almost without your noticing.

What sport should you take up? You may last have played at school and perhaps reacted against games because they were compulsory. Think again. As a pastime you might now enjoy a sport you hated then. Or you can try something new. Even if you already play something, why not give a different one a trial?

You may like ball games, whether football or netball, baseball or tennis—some people just seem to have more 'ball-sense' than others. Or you may prefer a sport such as riding or ice-skating. You may like involving yourself in team games such as basketball, or developing the individual skills of badminton. You may want the concentrated exercise of squash, or prefer the extended enjoyment of sailing. Whatever you like, the choice is up to you.

The following chart, a wide cross-section of various sports and games, gives you an indication of what each involves in terms of skill, equipment, the benefits you can gain, the facilities available and the social advantages you can expect. Whatever sport you adopt will require some initial effort—and probably some small cost. But the long-term benefits are great for your body, your personality, and your social scene.

You may feel wary because you have never played a particular sport before, thinking that you won't be able to play against people who have. Take your courage in your hands and you'll often be pleasantly surprised. Most people can reach a reasonable level of competence at any sport over a period of a few weeks—if you are persistent enough. Some people are extremely quick to pick up new sports, but even if you are not one of these people you can compensate with determination. To join some clubs, for example, you have to reach a certain level of skill.

All sports and games can be played at an organized level of competition or as a spontaneous get-together with your friends.

While nearly all games are good all-round exercises, some games offer specific benefits. If you want to lose weight take up an energetic sport, such as squash, football, badminton or basketball. It can be an enjoyable way to lose those extra inches. And you can make it a part of an overall exercise and diet programme: the wide variety of diets available and the exercises in this book will provide the components.

Most games and sports have one great advantage over many forms of 'static' exercises—they take you into the open air. This will help improve many aspects of your general health ranging from improved breathing to a better complexion.

Relaxation with friends is a natural part of most sports but it's more pronounced in some than in others. Frisbee, for example, is an ideal play-anywhere combination of leisure and sport, with no rules, no results, no restrictions. Other games offer relaxation in different ways. Golf, bowling, cricket, baseball and rounders don't demand your permanent and undivided attention. There will be gaps between your involvement where you can just relax and watch others playing. Some sports, like golf and ice-skating, can be played at exactly the pace you want to set. But all sports are intended to relax and refresh; and your first aim should always be to enjoy which one you become involved in.

Adaptability is a keynote to many of the sports listed in the chart. Most of them can be played at high competitive levels or as spontaneous get-togethers between friends. Football, for example, can be played in a serious league or as an unorganized kick-about; you can play a simple version of golf with just a putting club and a plastic tumbler in whatever space you can find; ten-pin bowling can be improvised with home-made skittles and rubber balls. You can even improve your level of fitness just by throwing a ball around. Such forms of improvized games are ideal if you feel that you're not fit or good enough to become involved in organized sport or that you don't have sufficient time to devote to them.

Today, with increasing leisure time, there's a great interest in sports. The facilities for amateur participation in sport are widespread and varied. Equipment is better and there is more choice in quality and price. The chance to learn and become involved in a sport is greater than ever before. More people are realizing that sport is an ideal way of spending those spare hours—keeping fit and healthy.

The following chart is a wide-ranging guide to different aspects of a cross-section of sports. It's intended to help you decide what each sport involves. Of course it can't be comprehensive—and you may like to search out sports it doesn't cover.

After you've decided which sport to take up check out the facilities available in your neighbourhood, the equipment you'll need and if there are some groups of people or clubs you can join. If you don't wish to use organized facilities but want the fun of playing a sport it's up to you to find a place. Get as many of your friends involved as possible. It will benefit them and make it more enjoyable for you.

BADMINTON

Badminton is played both indoors and outdoors on a court 44 feet long and 20 feet wide with wooden-framed rackets. The shuttlecock is put over a high net suspended 5 feet from the centre of the court. Each game runs to 15 points.

Facilities
Need a racket and a shuttlecock. A plastic shuttle is the cheapest and is up to standard. There are quite an amount of clubs which you can join. Fees are small and you should have no difficulty in joining. Badminton can be played all-year round either outside (if it's not too windy) or indoors.

Level of skill
Start at the bottom of the scale. The vital technique you need to learn is the wrist action. This is important to deception—a major part of the game—where you have to fool your opponent as to the type of shot, smash or delicate flick which you are going to play. Excellent for people who do not like ball games.

Benefits
Can be a very fast game, demanding delicacy of touch, lightning reflexes, suppleness and power of smash.

Number of people
Games are played in singles or doubles.

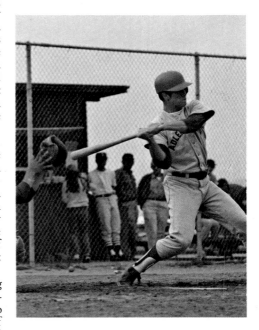

BASEBALL

Played with a round bat and a ball of rubber or cork covered with leather. Each fielder wears a leather glove or mitt on one hand. A game consists of nine innings: the time within which each team has a turn at bat. The team scoring most runs on a diamond-shaped pitch with three bases wins.

Facilities
Numerous facilities in the U.S.A. but is not played much in other countries, where other versions exist.

Level of skill
Does not require a high level of skill when played by amateurs, intent just on enjoyment rather than the competitive aspect. Like all games you will improve with practice.

Benefits
Demands speed, a sharp eye and good reflexes. If you play it frequently you can develop these qualities to a great extent. Like most team games, it can be played and enjoyed on a less organized level with friends.

Number of people
Played between two teams of nine players each. However, you can play with smaller teams by reducing the number of fielders and by decreasing the size of the boundaries.

BASKETBALL

Played on a court almost 100 feet long and 50 feet wide. Each team defends a basket, suspended at each end of the court. The ball, 30 inches in circumference, may be thrown, deflected by

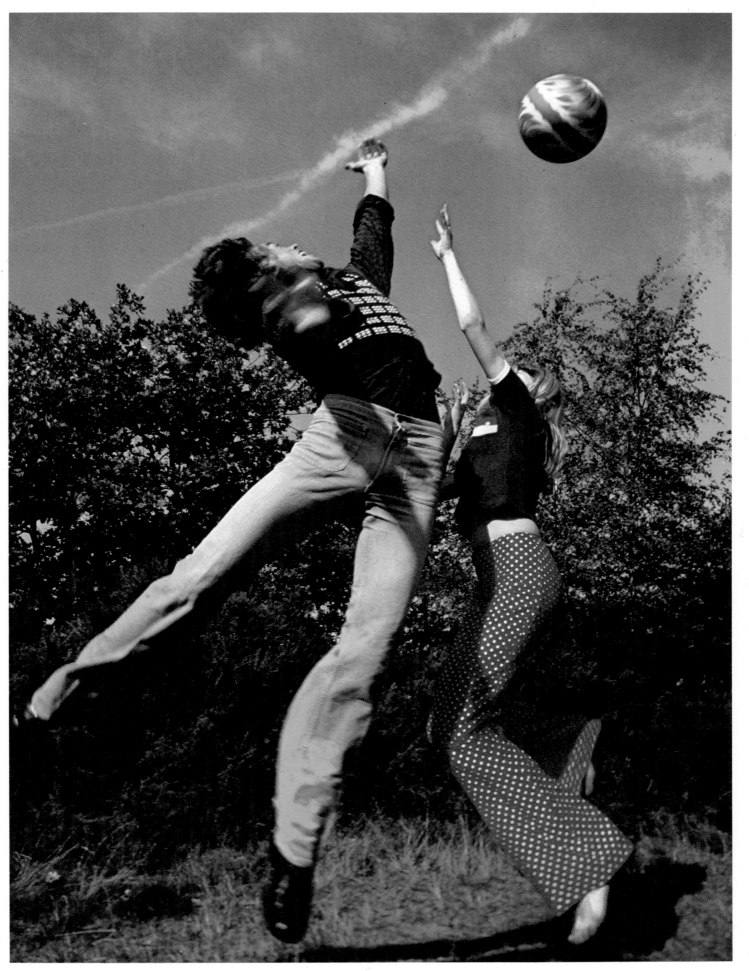

hand, rolled or dribbled in any direction within the confines of the court. A player scores two points each time he throws the ball into the basket from anywhere inside the court. A game consists of two 20-minute halves in Europe and 12-

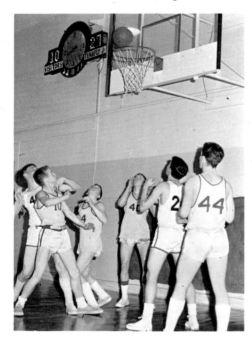

minute quarters in the U.S.A.

Facilities
No special equipment other than a pair of shorts, rubber-soled shoes and a singlet. A basketball is inexpensive. Plenty of public courts, both indoor and outdoor, available if you organize a two-team challenge with a group of friends. Not difficult to join a club where you can play regularly and more competitively. Can be played all the year round.

Level of skill
Played at most levels of skill, so you should find your own niche. You can move on to higher levels of competition after regular games have improved your ability.

Benefits
Calls for speed, sharpened reflexes and judgement. Improves concentration and reactions to other players' movements. Needs good team co-ordination.

Number of people
Two teams of 5 men each. If you can't find that number of people, just take a basketball to the nearest court and practice with two or three friends.

FOOTBALL
Soccer, Rugby League, Rugby Union, American Football, Canadian Football, Australian Rules

Facilities
Can be played on a regular weekly basis —with a team—or as an occasional work-out with friends in the park. (American football requires protective clothing). If playing occasionally a pair of tennis shoes, shorts and a ball are all you need.

Clubs for all types of football are numerous, and you should have no trouble in finding a team place at some level of skill.

You can arrange your own games with people at work or school and hire a pitch, splitting the cost between everybody.

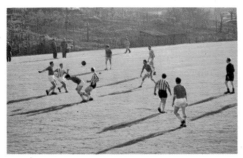

The hiring fee is usually minimal.

Level of skill
Can be played at all levels of skill. Play with opponents who are roughly the same standard as yourself to get more enjoyment. But go for riding, ice-skating, sailing, badminton and so on if your ball sense is weak.

Benefits
Improves most physical attributes—skill, stamina, reflexes, co-ordination, balance and acceleration. If you play with an organized team there are usually many club socials which you can attend. You can always ask to join in a park game to make up the number.

Number of people
Number needed to make up a soccer or American football team is 11, for rugby league 13, for rugby union 15, for Australian rules 18. However, un-organized and improvized games do not need the required number.

GOLF
Played on a 9-or-18-hole course. You can play either by shots (stroke-play) or by the number of holes won (match-play).

Facilities
Minimum number of clubs needed to play golf at a reasonable level is 7. The cost is likely to be relatively high, even if you can get a second-hand set. However, if you're really keen you can possibly get by with only 4 or 5 clubs. Numerous clubs in most countries. Many try to keep their membership to a certain number and so are usually difficult to join. Fees tend to be rather expensive, but there are public courses.

Level of skill
A reasonable level of skill is necessary, if only for the convenience of others using the course. You can get some practice in before applying for membership by using a driving range, a public park or a public course. The handicap system, used by most people playing golf, makes games very enjoyable and more fair.

Benefits
Walking in the fresh air is the main benefit, but it also develops your co-

ordination and balance and improves your powers of concentration. It's a casual, soothing and relaxing sport which nevertheless still involves friendly competitiveness.

Most clubs are centred round a club-house where socializing is easy. The yearly calendar is usually dotted with social events. Club competitions will enable you to meet and compete with other people. At some clubs the social life appears more important than the golf.

Number of people
Can play a round of golf alone, but it's more enjoyable if played with other people. Two or four is best.

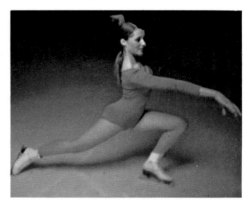

ICE-SKATING
Facilities
Skates, the only equipment needed, are relatively expensive to buy but you can hire them for a small fee.

Most towns and cities have rinks.

Level of skill
If you're starting from scratch prepare for a little embarrassment—you'll find it difficult to stay on your feet. Be persistent because you'll get the knack after an hour or so. Then it's practice makes perfect. Good for people with a sense of balance who aren't too good at ball games.

Benefits
Will greatly improve your balance and co-ordination, and is a good all-round form of exercise.

Most ice-rinks have bars and other amenities so that you can make it a social as well as a sporting occasion. Good for meeting the opposite sex.

Number of people
No limit to the amount of people you can skate with. The more people, the more fun. A mixture of good skaters and those who have never put feet on a rink will make for great enjoyment.

NETBALL
Similar to basketball, but usually played by women. The court—100 feet long by 50 feet—is divided into three zones, with players' movements restricted.

Facilities
Enjoys great popularity and you should-n't have any difficulty in joining a club or organizing your own games.

Level of skill
Played at all levels of skill. Try to play with people with a similar degree of proficiency.
Benefits
Requires good muscle control in twisting and jumping. Speed and accuracy are called for. Regular playing will develop these qualities.
Number of people
Each team consists of seven players.

be played by children. Of all ball games, it needs the least amount of ball sense.
Benefits
Plenty of fresh air and running. An ideal and easy way of spending a few hours with friends. The competitive element is small.
Number of people
Usually played by two teams of nine players each, but this is very flexible. Just alter the number of fielders.

little for tuition. Needs a good sense of co-ordination.
Benefits
One of the most exhilarating and rewarding of sports. Good exercise for all parts of the body and plenty of fresh air. Strong social side to sailing—and travel is inclusive.
Number of people
Varies with the size of the boat, from one to about eight.

SOFTBALL

Derived from baseball and played with a similar bat but a larger, softer ball. The rules are similar to baseball except that pitching is done underarm, and a game lasts for 7 innings.
Facilities
Except in the U.S.A. there are few softball clubs. Why not buy a bat and ball and organize your own games?
Level of skill
Generally needs a lower level of skill than baseball.
Benefits
As baseball.
Number of people
Softball requires two teams of nine players. But, like baseball, you can reduce the number of fielders.

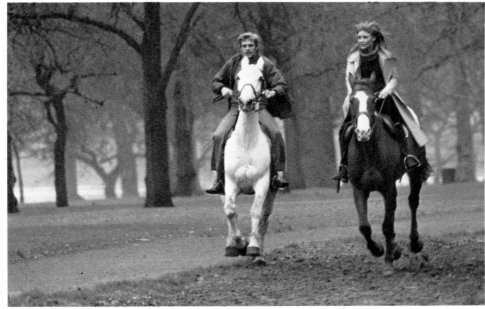

RIDING

Facilities
Most of us can't afford to keep a horse. Lessons are expensive but rewarding. The answer is often 'group ownership' and sharing.
Level of skill
Anyone can learn the basics with good tuition.
Benefits
Useful exercise and a very rewarding one. Riding schools and stables are good places for meeting people. If you compete in amateur races and hunts the social side is good.
Number of people
The number of people is almost irrelevant. Two people is probably the ideal.

ROUNDERS

The antecedent of baseball and softball, rounders is a very flexible game. Rules have always been elastic but basically they consist of bat striking ball and the strike running between five bases. Bases can be marked with clothes. The game is usually played with two innings for each team.
Facilities
Few organized facilities for rounders, but all you need is a large space, a bat and ball, and some friends.
Level of skill
No great skills are needed. Rounders can

SAILING

Facilities
Increasing in popularity all the time. The sea is best, but lakes and rivers can provide the facilities.
Boats vary from inexpensive small dinghies to ocean-going yachts.
Level of skill
It's easier to join a club to learn the basics on a small boat and then move to the size of boat which suits your taste. You can teach yourself but it's better to pay a

SQUASH

Squash is played on an enclosed four-walled court. The basic aim of each player is to hit the ball above a 19-inch-high strip on the front wall so that the opponent can not reach it with one bounce or cannot hit it back up against the front wall. The ball need not go directly from racket to back wall.
A game can last usually only about 15 minutes. Like badminton, you can only score with service.
Facilities
One of the world's fastest growing sports and demand often exceeds supply in courts. Because it's an indoor game it can be played all year round.

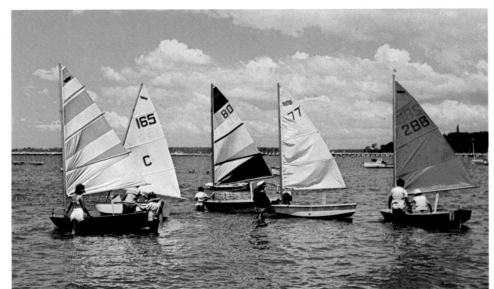

Squash demands tremendous stamina and concentration. It's best to start with someone a little better than you.

Benefits

Exhilarating and exhausting, squash will make you extremely fit and will enable you to lose some weight. It will sharpen your reflexes and build up your judgement and reactions. A good sport for getting the most exercise in a short time. Squash clubs normally have social facilities.

Squash is usually played in singles. Wait until you are proficient to play doubles because the pace is usually more hectic and the game complicated.

first player to reach 21 points with a 2-point lead wins the game.

A table tennis bat costs next to nothing. If you have the time or money you can easily make or buy your own table.

Facilities

Many clubs and halls for table tennis and you should have no difficulties in finding a place to play.

It might be more fun, if you have a large room and table, to play it at home, perhaps the garage.

Level of skill

One of the simplest of games and you can start playing without ever having played before.

can. You can also practice at home against a wall for the basic strokes.

Benefits

Improves your reflexes and co-ordination. If played frequently, you can lose weight. Increases your powers of concentration, suppleness and judgement. There is great opportunity for meeting people, both on and off the courts. Private tennis clubs usually have a number of social events.

Number of people

Played with two or four players. But, over a series of games, many of your friends can participate.

TENPIN BOWLING

The basic object of bowling is to knock down all 10 pins. Played on a wooden lane. The pins, numbered from one to ten, are 15 inches high. The distance over which the ball is bowled, from the front line to head pin -number 1) is 60 feet and the alley is 42 inches wide. There are gutters on each side of the lane. Bowling balls are 21 inches in circumference and are usually made of hard rubber. It has three finger holes for the thumb, middle and ring fingers.

Facilities

Large number of bowling centres. You just go along, pay a fee for a bowling lane and hire a pair of bowling shoes. Being indoor, it's an all-year sport.

Level of skill

Best to play your first few games with someone who is fairly proficient and who knows the rules and scoring.

Benefits

Above all a relaxing sport. It also improves balance, develops poise and cultivates co-ordination and concentration. Good for legs, back and arms.

Most bowling centres have bars and cafes. In some, hundreds of people can play at once. Good for meeting the opposite sex.

Number of people

The maximum number of people for a game is five. More can play but it can be restrictive.

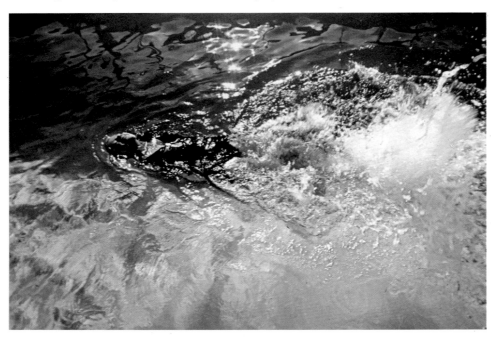

SWIMMING

Facilities

Perhaps the easiest of all the major sports to adopt. Pools are plentiful (outdoor and indoor) and most people are near enough the sea to take advantage of it.

Level of skill

Once a basic stroke (probably the breast-stroke) is mastered, you can move on to the other three. And to diving. Swimming is also an essential skill for you to learn. You can always join a club and, if you're good, go on to water-skiing, skin-diving etc.

Benefits

The best all-round exercise you can get, utilising all the body's muscles and joints. By the sea or by a pool, it's a great way to meet people of both sexes.

Number of people

Endless, but it's always better with a group of friends with whom you can enjoy the swimming—and splashing.

TABLE TENNIS

Played indoors with rubber-covered bats and a celluloid ball. The table is 9-feet long and 5-feet wide. A net 6-inches high is stretched across the middle. The

Benefits

Will improve you concentration and judgement. Though not particularly energetic it's one of the few games you can play in the home which involves movement.

Level of skill

Good family game. Singles or doubles.

TENNIS

Played (usually outdoors) on a court measuring 78 feet long and 27 feet wide. Courts are asphalt or grass. Tennis is played with wood or steel-framed rackets used by the players to hit the ball above a net into the opponents half of the court.

Facilities

All you need is a racket and a minimum of two balls. Because of rapid wear and tear, new balls will be needed frequently, but they are inexpensive. Courts can be private or public. The cost of membership to a private club is usually reasonable and will save you a great amount of inconvenience; but public courts are numerous and usually easy to book.

Level of skill

Can be enjoyed at any level of skill. But obviously it will become more enjoyable as you get better. Practice as much as you

All About Exercise Machines

When a person considers buying an exercise machine, or using one in a gym, he or she often thinks, It costs a lot, so it must be good. Up to a point, that is true. A neat, well-made piece of equipment can be a great incentive to exercise.

Yet, no matter how faithfully the instructions are followed, and how diligently the exercise is carried out, the person using the machine may well be labouring under a false impression. He or she may have made a bad buy. This is not due to an inaccurate brochure or a fast-talking salesman, but because of lack of knowledge about both the machines and individual requirements.

What, then, are the factors that should determine the choice of an exercise machine? In terms of all-round physical fitness, there are three main considerations. The first is mobility. Does the equipment permit the joints and muscles of the body to move over their full potential range? The second factor is strength. Does the machine develop the muscle tone and power necessary to cope with movements against resistance in all ranges and directions? And the third consideration is cardio-vascular efficiency. To what extent does the equipment make the heart and lungs work at a higher than normal rate without stress, and how much does it increase the rate of recovery after exertion? Each of these fitness factors contribute to endurance and the reduction of fatigue.

As well as these central considerations when choosing an exercise machine, there are other, more practical points. These include the initial cost of the apparatus, the cost of running and repairing it, the attractiveness and portability of the equipment, the amount of time involved in its use and the effort it requires in relation to the results it produces.

Many exercise machines sell not on the basis of their contribution to improving general fitness but on their claims, theoretical or proved, to be an effective method of reducing weight. But, no matter how complicated the machine, and how determinedly and regularly it is used, one simple fact must be kept in mind—weight reduction can only be effectively achieved with dieting.

While this can be aided by general and regular exercise, it is impossible to lose weight by doing nothing and letting a machine do the work. However it is possible, with only exercise, or using some exercise machines, to lose inches as opposed to weight. Unfortunately, many people turn to exercise machines in the hope of an easy solution to their weight problems. They are nearly always disappointed.

Machines for exercise vary widely in size, application, results and cost.

Rowing Machines

There are three main types of rowing machines. The principle of all of them is the same. The feet are braced and the body slides forward on a seat as the oars are pulled back. In some rowing machines the resistance to be overcome is provided by rubber or steel cables, but in the more expensive models hydraulic pressure is used.

In terms of general fitness, rowing machines make a great demand on the major muscles groups of the legs, arms, back and hips and create a high rate of activity for the heart and lungs. Used regularly and properly, general endurance can be greatly improved.

Increased muscular endurance, however, is obviously confined to the groups of muscles being exercised, and then only over a fairly limited range. The same can be said of the ability of rowing machines to develop muscular strength. While they have an effect on specific areas of the body, they lack the adaptability to exercise other muscle groups over any sort of effective range. Loss of inches, particularly around the waist, can be achieved if the machine is used regularly and vigorously. The more expensive rowing machines have a mechanism for adjusting the resistance provided in either the seat or the oars.

The rubber cables lose their tension more quickly than those made of steel, but they can be easily replaced. The hydraulically-controlled machines, although considerably more expensive, are probably worth the money if the machine is seriously used as an aid to physical fitness. But a rowing machine can only be used at home. It's not the kind of exercise equipment you take away for weekends, on holiday or on a business trip.

Static Cycles

Static cycles, bicycles which do not move, vary from very simple models which have just a frame and a wheel, to those that are more sophisticated, with adjustable seats and resistance gauges and meters. Nearly all types of static cycles have resistance applied to the wheel either in the form of a block brake or, more often, a band which operates like a fan-belt on a car engine. The models that have larger wheels, with the resistance applied to about two-thirds of the circumference, are normally the most effective. With the block type of resistance, even if it is adjustable, there is not the same degree of friction or consistency of resistance, and movement can become jerky.

The cycle is good for toning and strengthening the muscles in the legs and hips, and for the improvement of endurance in these areas, even though the range over which those muscles operate is limited. And for increasing the efficiency of the heart and lungs, this is one of the best pieces of exercise equipment available. Because it concentrates on the legs, however, it has little to offer those people who want to improve their all-round mobility or strength.

Combined with a sensible reducing diet, exercising several times a week for 10 to 15 minutes on the cycle against sufficient resistance can produce reasonable results. And those who use it faithfully report a great loss of inches, particularly from the thighs.

One of the advantages of a good static cycle is that the resistance is adjustable. As you become more fit, you can increase the resistance. You can also measure the "speed" you are doing and the "distance" you cover. On the negative side, and on a practical level, is the cost of a static cycle and the difficulty of transporting it. In addition, it is necessary to seek advice on a programme for its use since few cycles are accompanied by useful instructions.

Chest Expanders

Chest expanders are based either on rubber or, more commonly, steel cables. Although they have a much wider range of use, in terms of muscles and joints

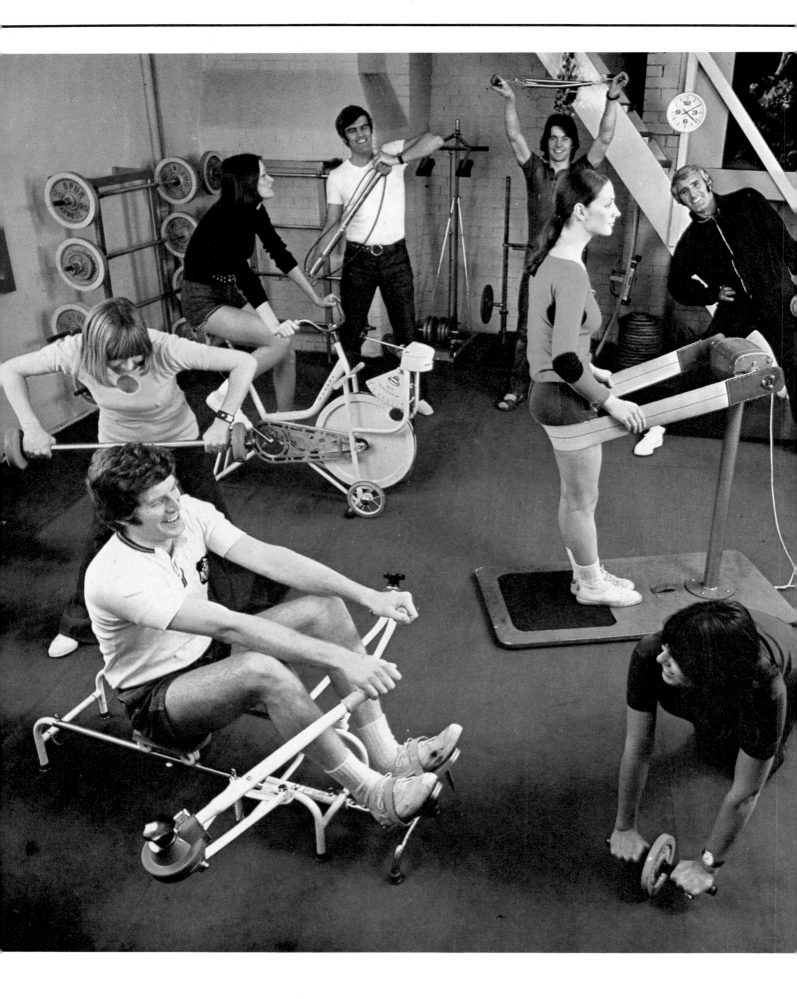

which can be exercised, than their more expensive cousins, the rowing machines, they are most effective when used to exercise the arms and shoulders. The trunk and legs can be exercised, but only with limited success compared to the benefits to the upper body.

Because of their wider range, chest expanders are more valuable than either rowing machines or static cycles for increasing joint mobility. If they are used on a regular basis to their full potential and with some enthusiasm, a slight increase in cardio-vascular efficiency will result, and the number of calories burned up can be quite high. In addition, they are cheap, versatile and highly portable.

It is as well, however, to be aware of the limitations of chest expanders. Although the word "chest" should not be taken literally, since other parts of the body, particularly the limbs, may well be involved, many benefits that may seem to be derived from their use may be deceptive. Some instructions, for example, recommend that knee-bends be done holding a position with the expanders across the chest. The resulting strength in the legs will be nothing to do with the expanders—the same results would have been achieved with the arms at the sides. It is not unusual for the instructions which accompany all types of apparatus which involve springs, cables or compression to include exercises which in no way depend on the equipment for their effectiveness.

Resistance Exercisers
Resistance exercisers differ. *Bullworker 2*, which employs steel cables on the archery principle, allows a greater range of movement than that provided by chest expanders. Once the individual's limit of compression or extension is reached, the isometric principle of fixed muscular contraction comes into play. Due to their limited range, isometrics are not suitable for the development of mobility, but they are useful for strengthening specific muscle groups. The cardio-vascular element is practically negligible for all resistance exercisers.

Like chest expanders, resistance exercisers use up some extra energy and can be helpful in slimming. The "power meter" on the *Bullworker 2* has a competitive appeal and if the instructions are carefully followed this exerciser should strengthen men's muscles and improve their shape.

Vibrator Belts
Vibrator belts are sold as a short cut to spot-reduction, but most of the claims made for them are totally unjustified. The indisputable principle of slimming —cutting down on the intake of calories by dieting and increasing the output of calories by exercise—is openly defied. Standing with a throbbing belt around one part of the anatomy can help a person to relax, particularly at the end of an exercise session, but it uses up no more energy, and therefore no more calories, than if the person were just standing doing nothing. There is no evidence to show that mechanical massage can have any effect in breaking down fat. Vibrator belts have no value in increasing mobility, strength or endurance—and they are quite expensive.

Many users of such equipment, particularly women, stay on the machines for too long in the mistaken belief that they will lose inches. Research has shown that this can damage blood cells in the areas being vibrated and the time on each part of the body—if the user is determined to stay with it—should be limited to a few minutes.

Artificial Exercisers
Electrical stimulation to produce muscle contraction and relaxation has been used for many years and, as part of rehabilitation programmes, is one of the main methods used to strengthen muscles which have wasted away to such an extent that the patient finds it difficult to use them. Pads are put next to the skin. The pads are connected by wires to a power unit, and electrical impulses passing through the muscles cause them to contract. Over a period of time, using many such contractions, the muscle gradually strengthens and becomes accustomed to its role.

Aside from physiotherapy, however, there is little that can be achieved by these machines for the average person. This is further accentuated by the considerations of the time recommended for their use, which is extensive, and the cost. The machines are very expensive to buy and the alternative is a regular course of treatment, also not cheap, at a special centre.

If a person's muscles are flabby and his level of fitness exceptionally low, then the muscle tone can be improved by the use of such a machine. But the machines in no way improve general physical condition.

Courses which involve electrical muscle stimulation often recommend and outline a diet and it is the following of the diet, rather than the time spent on the machine, which is responsible for the achievement of the greatest results.

Weights
Because of their adjustable size and weight, barbells and dumb-bells can be used by men and women, old and young, and by those people who are fit as well as those who are out of condition. It is this versatility, often not appreciated by people who consider weight-lifting to be strenuous and good only for muscle building, which makes this type of exercise equipment so useful.

Most free exercises, which allow natural joint movement and have few limitations, can be done with weights to suit particular resistance. General fitness can be considerably improved by doing many repetitions of one exercise with light resistance on a regular basis, and this in turn exercises and develops the heart and lungs. Different positions with varying weights and repetitions can produce muscular strength and endurance, and since all joints can be exercised over their full range, greater mobility is almost inevitable.

The expenditure of calories can be high during vigorous exercise—high repetitions with light weights.

Weights are expensive to buy and are difficult to transport. But they are a lasting investment. There is no cost involved in their use, they never need repair and this is the only form of exercise equipment that can be gradually built up over a period of time.

Exercise Wheels
It is nearly always the one-movement type of exercise equipment that fascinates and attracts the greatest number of people. The success of the exercise wheels, which almost reached craze proportions in the late 1960's, reflect the desire of the public to get fit with the minimum expenditure of energy.

The hula-hoop, which preceded the wheel and had an even bigger following, is another example Here the accent of movement was more obviously centred on the waist and hips—and any apparatus with a possibility of reducing the waistline has an instant and wide appeal.

The exercise wheel is no exception. It is an excellent and relatively cheap piece of equipment for strengthening the stomach muscles and those which cross the front of the hips and, to a lesser extent, the chest and back muscles. But its value ends here, except for the weighted wheels which come with a chart that tells the purchaser about other exercises they can perform with it for different muscles.

Most of the wheels, however, recommend the same basic exercise. Kneeling on the floor, the wheel is used to push forward as far as is comfortable before going back to the starting position. When using the wheel the back must be kept straight and the buttocks well up to avoid the chance of injury. It is imperative not to overstretch and to build up very gradually with the wheel.

No exercise equipment will give you much benefit if you don't use it regularly and for sufficiently long sessions. And it is expensive. A static cycle, for instance, is an expensive way to exercise when you consider that an ordinary bicycle can be picked up cheaply secondhand, and moreover it will give you excellent outdoor exercise *and* get you places too. So consider carefully what your particular needs are and whether you will have the perseverance to use your exercise equipment regularly before you take the plunge.

The chart on the following pages gives you a useful summary of the value of all these machines.

	Rowing Machines			Static Cycles	Chest Expanders	
Key ★ poor ★★ fair ★★★ good ★★★★ very good ★★★★★ excellent S for specific muscle groups only C continuous payment usually necessary P private instruction and supervision necessary	rubber cables	steel cables	hydraulic pressured			
All-round mobility	★	★	★	★	★★	
General fitness	★★	★★	★★★	★★★★	★★	
Muscular endurance	S ★★★	S ★★★★	S ★★★	S ★★★★	S ★★★	
Strength	S ★★	S ★★	S ★★	S ★★★	S ★★★	
Muscle tone	S ★★	S ★★	S ★★	S ★★	S ★★★	
Weight reduction	★★	★★	★★	★★★	★	
Adaptability	★	★	★	★	★★★	
Multi-purpose value	★	★	★	★	★★	
Specific or limited value	★★	★★	★★★	★★★★	★★★	
Durability	★★	★★	★★★	★★★	★★★	
Portability	★	★	★	★	★★★★★	
Books or instructions	★	★	★	★	★★★	

Resistance Exercisers	Vibrator Machines	Artificial Exercisers	Weights	Exercise Wheels
★★			★★★	★
★★			★★★★	★
S ★★★★			★★★★	S ★★★
S ★★★★		★	★★★★★	S ★★★
S ★★★★		★★★	★★★★★	S ★★
★			★★★	★
★★★			★★★★	
★★			★★★★	★
★★★	★	★★★	★★★★	★★★
★★★	★★★	C	★★★★★	★★★
★★★★	★		★	★★★
★★★	★	P	★★★	★★

Keep fit and live longer

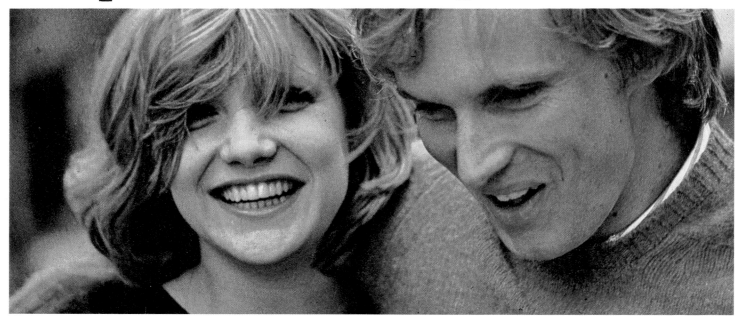

Your health is in your own hands. Fitness and health are your birthright, so safeguard them well, and you can enjoy a fuller and happier life.

If you've been following any of the exercise programmes in this book regularly, you will have noticed an improvement in your overall health, more vitality, and a general feeling of wellbeing. Other people have probably noticed it too.

Keeping fit is a matter of commonsense, and many, though of course not all, of the factors which affect your health are within your own control. You can tell if your posture is incorrect without help from a doctor, and you know there is a lot you can do to put things right. Unless quite early in life you establish good postural habits, correcting deeply-ingrained faults will become progressively more difficult. But never despair—you can put yourself back on the right track at any age.

Exercise is of prime importance. You may well have no intention of doing anything violent, but regular exercise is still vital, even to everyday living. You can offset the normal ageing processes by keeping your body trim and fit. Much of the incentive to do this must come from within yourself. Being able to walk up that mountain when you want to, or run for a bus, and stay younger longer as a result—that makes health worthwhile. If this is not sufficient incentive to you, remember that life itself is sweet and worth making the most of until the very end. So make a habit of regular exercise for a longer and happier life.

If you can possibly help it, don't ever carry an extra pound of weight. The pleasures of food and drink are very seductive and the longer you live, the longer you will be able to enjoy them. The discomfort of an overweight body reduces your mobility, and declining mobility tends to make you console yourself with food. A vicious circle is established—one which you can only escape from by adhering to sensible eating habits combined with regular exercise.

The evidence of damage to your health from cigarette smoking is all too clear. There is not just the higher risk of lung cancer, but bronchitis and other ailments. So if you must smoke, do so in moderation: better not to smoke at all.

Moderation in all things is an old-fashioned but thoroughly sensible maxim. If you grow up with good eating habits you are less likely to suffer the miseries of overweight in later life. And if you take regular exercise as a matter of course then you won't need to rush into a strenuous exercise programme to get fit in time for your summer holidays —perhaps pulling a muscle or straining your back in the process. Similarly, everyone needs regular work and regular relaxation. Modern living inevitably involves a lot of stress and it is only sensible to minimize it by putting work right out of your mind when you relax, and getting away from it all completely once in a while. It's a wise man who knows his limitations and orders his life within those limits. You're better off as a live chief clerk than as a dead managing director!

It's obvious that to achieve these thoroughly worthwhile aims, self-control is needed and that is certainly no bad thing. But like everything which controls human behaviour, good habits are best acquired when you are young.

Lastly, don't get obsessed with health, fitness and exercise to the point where it becomes just another neurosis. Follow sensible rules—be concerned about them—and good and golden health will be yours throughout life.

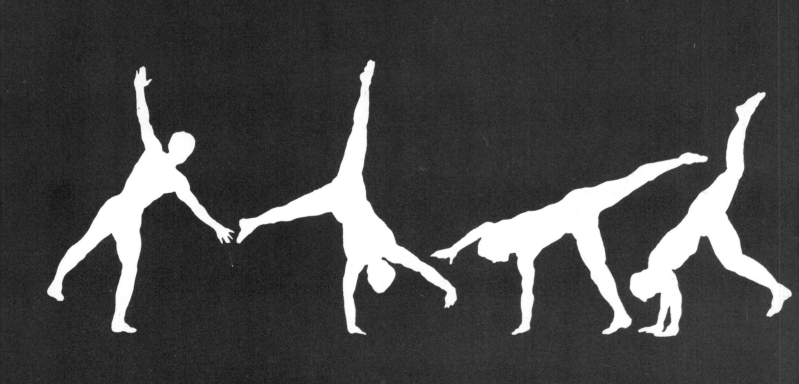